Advance P
Confidence Thr

A great book! It is so touching and inspirational to see the love and passion for the work that Jerry does in helping others to become all that they are capable of being. It is written in the common man's language with great analogies and examples from his own life experiences as well as the example(s) of others. It is an excellent book, an easy read while still being very detailed, based on the science of nutrition, exercise and exercise physiology. And, of course, including the importance of the role that God should play in every aspect of our lives only adds to the substance of the book.
~Pete Boudreaux, National Coach of the Year and National High School Hall of Fame

We all long to live a healthy lifestyle where we are strong in mind and body. Jerry lays out the practical but necessary tools that are needed to accomplish these goals. Confidence Through Health covers every aspect of physical and mental fitness, for both the seasoned athlete and the overweight or unhealthy individual. We all can live a full, abundant life and Jerry shows us how to train ourselves to fully engage in that life.
~Pam Moorhead, MS, Owner of Health and Soul Fitness

Jerry Snider has written a must-read for anyone wanting to make a meaningful lifestyle change. He masterfully combines the fundamentals of health and wellness with living a faith-filled God-centered life. This book has uncovered the lies I was telling myself about what to eat and how to exercise. Now I can see where I need healthy changes and have simple and practical tools to make it happen.
~ Jennifer Snyder, Professional Organizer

Confidence Through Health is an excellent source of answers for the issues facing most of us today. How to eat healthily and maintain a healthy lifestyle while dealing with our day-to-day challenges. It's an easy read full of great information. Very inspiring to get on the right path to healthy eating and exercise. The book inspired me to get back on the right track and I loved the biblical references.
~Jeanne Rieger, former client

CONFIDENCE THROUGH HEALTH

Live the Healthy Lifestyle God Designed

Good planning and hard work lead to prosperity,
but hasty shortcuts lead to poverty.
– Proverbs 21:5

By Jerry Snider

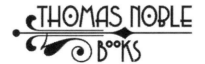

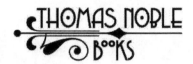

Author Contact: AllinHealthandWellness.com

Author photo by Laura LeBlanc of Laura LeBlanc Photography

Thomas Noble Books

Wilmington, DE

www.thomasnoblebooks.com

Library of Congress Control Number: 2018943449

ISBN: 978-1-945586-10-1

First Printing: 2018

Editing by Gwen Hoffnagle

Cover Design by Sarah Barrie of Cyanotype.ca

This book is dedicated to my wife and best friend Jenny Snider. The joy you bring to my life is indescribable. There is nothing I would rather do in this world than spend time with you. I thank God every day for creating you and I look forward to years of happiness together.

To my children Abigail and Tai - always know that with God all things are possible.

TABLE OF CONTENTS

INTRODUCTION
MY STORY

*For we are God's masterpiece. He has created us anew
in Christ Jesus, so we can do the good things he planned
for us long ago.*
– Ephesians 2:10

Let me state the obvious: my story is not your story. One thing we can all agree on is everyone's story is different. This makes it difficult emotionally if your main goal is to lose weight or enhance your health, because someone you know might have huge success with a particular health plan while you get nothing from it.

I was blessed with a great metabolism. Please don't hate me. As Jenny, my wife, says, "Jerry can just think about losing weight and he does." Of course that's not true. Even with a fast metabolism it takes planning and effort to live a healthy lifestyle. As I will explain in this book, a healthy lifestyle is more than just a low number on the scale. I grew up very active in sports – soccer, water skiing, cross country, and track – not to mention all the sports I played for fun in the neighborhood.

Early Sports Years

Through my elementary school years I became very successful in soccer, culminating in eighth grade when my team won the Louisiana State Championship and traveled to compete at the USA U14 Regional Championships in Florida. While we did not fare too well in that tournament, I vividly remember having an assist off a corner kick.

In high school I was discovered as a runner during a 12-minute run test in my physical education class in the fall of freshman year. One of the other kids in class told me I should try cross country. While soccer was still my overall plan, I loved to run and thought, "Why not?" It turned out to be a very good decision. I played for the junior varsity soccer team in high school as a freshman, but I wasn't too fond of the coaches, and it turned out that was the last year I played soccer. I competed in track with some success at the end of my freshman year. Then my first experience with weight gain occurred that summer of 1989.

I grew up with four siblings and we often took turns spending time in the summer with our grandparents. That summer my younger brother and I stayed with them for something like six or eight weeks. Grandmothers are great, except when they allow you to eat an entire box of Twinkies® *every day*! Yep, in appreciation for helping my Papaw out with his projects she bought me Twinkies. Needless to say, except for a bit of water skiing there was no true exercise or sports training going on that summer.

I returned to high school to start my sophomore year and found I had gained over 20 pounds that summer. I weighed in at over 150 pounds, which is a lot considering

I graduated from high school at 135 pounds. I was nicknamed "Doughboy" by the team. Not exactly my finest sports moment. It didn't stop me though, because I knew I could accomplish something through running. By the end of that season I was selected as the last runner of the seven-member team that would compete at state. I turned in the race of my life to that point, placing 13th at state while running second on my team. And we won the team title that year.

I don't remember saying this but my mom will tell you that at that meet I told her I would win a state title before I graduated from high school. In my senior year I did just that, winning the Louisiana 5A State Cross Country title, Indoor 1500m title, and Outdoor 3200m title. I used my success at running to attain a scholarship to run cross country and track at Texas A&M University.

My running career at A&M was a bit of a roller coaster. I dealt with a few injuries from season to season but luckily none were too serious. I showed promise, but looking back I'll admit I let distractions get in the way of reaching my true running potential. One of the most memorable experiences was running anchor leg on the 4x1500m relay at Penn Relays in 1996. I finished my collegiate career as a three-year letterman and have medals from both the Southwest Conference and the Big XII Conference meets.

My Life's Purpose Revealed

While I was at A&M, my grandmother went into the hospital for quadruple bypass surgery. Heart surgery is nothing to mess with, and within 24 hours she was in surgery again for a bowel resection. Not something typical.

Not something an elderly woman who did not exercise was physically prepared for, either.

I vividly remember that it was not a fun experience to witness my grandmother suffering in the hospital. During that time I decided to focus my studies on exercise physiology. I did not want anyone else to have to see their grandmother in the hospital for heart issues that are very preventable.

About six months later she passed away. It was the spring of 1996, and to that point I had my sights set on trying to make the Olympic Trials for track. But I did not really recover emotionally that track season. I was just a few seconds off the qualifying time, which seems close but a few seconds is a lot in the 1500m. That is God's plan, so I am okay with it – one of those times in life when you set a goal, do not achieve it, and move on to the next goal.

I went on to finish my college running career and met my future wife, Jenny, doing an internship in cardiac rehabilitation. Jenny is also an exercise physiologist. What I learned in that internship is that she has a talent for working with the elderly and with recovering patients, and that is not my forte. I am much more suited to working with those who want to prevent cardiac disease and for those whose goal is athletic performance. So I went into the business world because I am the second of five kids and Mom and Dad wanted me off their dime.

I Should Have Known Better

Over time I stopped regular exercise, stopped maintaining a healthy diet, and lived without a genuine plan for my health. Even though I knew far better, I let life dictate my health.

Fast-forward to 2015, and I had finally had enough. I had gained a good 40 pounds since college. It was time to do something. Three things instigated the change. First, God told me to start a business focused on helping people get healthy. I had the schooling for it. I had the desire for it. And now I had the business experience to know how to go out on my own as a business owner. But I would have to start living a healthy lifestyle again, which meant a regular exercise routine and eating healthy foods.

Next was my children. Having adopted both of our kids, it was a struggle just to start our family (which is a whole different story I might write someday). Our kids were four and five years old at the time. I was finding it difficult to play with them because it was hard to keep up. My knees, hips, and muscles simply did not want to do what my mind told them to do. I knew regular exercise and stretching would help me regain my flexibility and strength.

The third thing was vanity. I was wearing size 36 pants and they were starting to get tight. I know some of you would kill to fit into a size 36, but I had graduated from college wearing a size 28. Emotionally I just could not let myself – a former track star, educated in ways to stay healthy – move to a 10-inch-bigger size.

So change happened. Beginning on August 1st of 2015 I changed my life. I started slow and steady, along the way developing the program I now use for my clients. By January 1st of 2016 I was down 30 pounds. I began training to become a life coach and was certified by the end of March of 2016. I already had the knowledge of health and fitness along with a degree to back it up, but I knew that true transformation to a healthy lifestyle involves more than just a diet change or an exercise routine. I launched my business in the spring of 2016 and set my first big athletic goal since college: run a marathon in December of 2016.

Even though I knew there would be stumbling blocks along the way, I had no idea how big one of those blocks would be.

Did Not See That Coming

July 14th, 2016 – a date I will never forget. It was a Thursday. We were on our annual camping/waterskiing vacation with extended family. In my refurbished, healthy body, I decided to do something I had never done before. I had been waterskiing on my own since the age of seven, and my mom carried me as she skied when I was an infant. I could slalom at competitive speeds. I had ridden trick skis since I was 10. I had ridden shoe skis, wakeboards, backwards slalom, and a ski skat (a slalom ski literally two feet long). I had barefooted once. Having this wealth of experience and a body that was stronger than it had been in 20 years... why not try a trick on skis I had never done before?

As we made a pass by camp, I skied outside the wake on the right side. I threw the rope behind my back and prepared for a 360 spin. I had done this probably 100 times or more in my life, but for the first time I attempted to do the trick I had dreamed of doing but never had the guts for: I turned towards the wake and went full force into an attempt at a wake helicopter, jumping the wake and doing the 360 in the air.

This story would have no relevance if I had not fallen, right? Yep, and it was a hard fall. I had fallen hard before.

Back as a teen I had fallen riding the ski skat. My heels touched the back of my head and I thought I had broken my back. Thankfully I did not. I also fell once making a turn on slalom at 36 mph and skipped across the lake, separating a rib.

Something about this fall was instantly different. I started screaming before I even came out of the water. Later I couldn't understand how I had not drowned because I know my mouth was wide open underwater, screaming. I rolled over in the water and looked at my left knee and ankle. My knee was visually out of place, and by the way the ski was floating it appeared that I had broken my ankle. Other than screaming for help, my first reaction was, "How am I going to get out of the water?" Thankfully it happened right in front of camp because I had planned to land the trick and be a show-off.

It turned out that the binding on the ski had torn a little bit so there was no issue with my ankle. But then my attention went to my knee and I had to push my lower leg back into alignment so my knee would look normal. I knew instantly that I had torn my medial collateral ligament (MCL). Once back at camp, which included a trip on a makeshift water stretcher (did you know that floaties have an emergency medical use?), I messaged my doctor back home. I told him to go ahead and get the MRI scheduled because this was bad.

The MRI revealed not just a grade 3 MCL tear but a completely ruptured posterior cruciate ligament (PCL). There was also plenty of other minor damage. Thankfully nothing needed surgery, but the surgeon said no running until January at the earliest. At first I told him that wouldn't work because I had a race to run in December. He laughed and told me not to be crazy.

Sorry, but I am a little crazy. Anyone who has competed in track and field will tell you that pole-vaulters are the craziest athletes of the sport, followed by long-distance runners. I believe 100 percent in the power of mind over matter. I also know what the human body is capable of if you decide you want to achieve it. Knowing the full marathon would be too difficult given the time I had for recovery, I changed my race registration to the half marathon. After several physical therapy sessions, months in a knee brace, and lots of my own home therapy, I was running on a treadmill just three months after the injury – *not* waiting until January. And with just 11 weeks of running under my belt I competed in the BCS Half-Marathon in College Station, Texas. I placed third in my age group and 60th overall out of over 1,800 runners.

Because I had raced wearing my knee brace, during the ride home I asked Jenny if she thought it was a legitimate third place – I had gotten help from an apparatus. She laughed and thought (and still thinks) I was nuts because I did it with only three of four ligaments in my knee.

It is also worth mentioning that I have suffered from a spontaneous pneumothorax – collapsed lung – twice (in July of 2011 and September of 2013). Both times my right lung collapsed while I was sleeping. To this day I wake up at times wondering if it has collapsed again. While it should not collapse again because it has been basically glued to my rib cage, you just never know. But I run on, knowing what does not kill me makes me stronger.

So that is me. I am a husband, a father, an exercise physiologist, an athlete, a certified life coach, a sports performance coach, a business owner, and apparently now a writer.

Why This Book?

While I readily admit that my weight and health challenges are not as dire as those that many people face, I understand struggles to overcome challenges. Remember, I was called Doughboy for several years. I still cringe when I see a Pillsbury commercial. But what is more important than the size of the challenge is that a lot of incorrect information about how to become healthier appears in the media and in advertising. It's hard to know what information to trust – what is true and correct versus simply a ploy to make a profit.

My goal in writing *Confidence Through Health* is to help you develop a healthy lifestyle by changing your mindset about food and exercise. We all know habits are hard to break. You are not a picky eater; you have simply developed a habit of eating the same types of foods. What you eat at one meal has a direct effect on what you crave afterwards. This is what gets you into trouble if you don't plan your meals.

Can your habit be so strong that it becomes an addiction? Sure it can. Can addictions be beaten? YES! Your addiction to sweets, soda, chips, or anything else can be beaten; just ask any former smoker or recovering alcoholic. The difference is that you can live without tobacco or alcohol – in fact your health gets better without them; but you cannot live without food for very long. This is why food addictions can be overwhelming and hard to deal with.

Food addictions are self-created. Eating certain types of foods, often from an early age, trains your body to crave those foods. If you purposefully decide to eat other types of foods, your body then becomes addicted to those new foods. You might assume I'm referring to being addicted to unhealthy foods, but this goes for both unhealthy and healthy foods. Someone who has been following a healthy meal plan for years can very easily become addicted to fruits, vegetables, and other nutrient-rich foods. Becoming addicted to healthy foods is a lifestyle change you should strive for.

When you feed your body, the food is broken down and the nutrients are used as energy, or fuel. The first step in understanding how to eat healthy is to understand that you are fueling your body. Food is fuel, plain and simple. Transforming the way you think about the food you eat will have a bigger impact on your transition to healthy eating than anything else you do.

CHAPTER 1

OUR DECLINING HEALTH

My son, pay attention to what I say; turn your ear to my words. Do not let them out of your sight, keep them within your heart; for they are life to those who find them and health to one's whole body.

— Proverbs 4:20-22

How Did We Get Here?

According to the Centers for Disease Control and Prevention's (CDC) National Center for Health Statistics, in 2014, 70.7 percent of Americans over the age of 20 were overweight or obese. (https://www.cdc.gov/nchs/fastats/obesity-overweight.htm) (I'll call it 70 percent from here forward for simplicity). It's obvious from that high percentage that the weight-control piece of a healthy lifestyle is so much more than a basic formula of eating and exercise. While I didn't look unhealthy at my heaviest weight, I was over 15 pounds above what is considered a healthy body mass index (BMI). (A healthy BMI, which is a calculation based on your height and weight, is between 18.5 and 25.) I was also 30 to 35 pounds above the ideal weight for my height. Even with all my training, I fell victim to the trends in our society. But it does not have to be that way, and I am proof of that. (The CDC considers those with a BMI between 25 and 29.9 to be overweight and those with a BMI of 30 or higher to be obese.) (https://www.cdc.gov/ncbddd/disabilityandhealth/obesity.html)

Think about that 70 percent of Americans with a BMI over 25 for a minute. If you are from a family of three, two of you are overweight or obese. Think about your extended family, your coworkers, your fellow church members. That statistic means that in a church with 100 members only 30 of them are at a healthy weight.

With the trends of the last few years, I am fearful this statement from the CDC's Bob Anderson, Chief of the Mortality Statistics Branch at the CDC's National Center for Health Statistics, will come true:

> If we're not careful, we could end up with declining life expectancy for three years in a row, which we haven't seen since the Spanish flu, 100 years ago. (http://www.cnn.com/2017/12/21/health/us-life-expectancy-study/index.html)

There are at least three causes for this trend: One is a shift away from industrialization and towards technology and customer service, which require less physical activity on the part of our workforce. The other two are a poor diet – specifically the unhealthy fast-food diet, and lack of exercise.

Our work environment is an important factor in this trend. There are far more desk jobs than in decades past, so there are fewer people working manual jobs that require physical energy. And in case you haven't heard this yet, a sedentary lifestyle such as sitting at a desk for eight hours a day is not good for your health.

But there are countries all over the world that have moved into the technology age without the weight issues of Americans. And there are plenty of Americans who have desk jobs who still find a way to live a healthy lifestyle, though they are clearly in the minority. The jobs themselves are not the problem; the challenge is to change our eating habits to fit this more sedentary lifestyle. Similarly, there are many former athletes who still eat like they are in training even though they are no longer competing. Without the continued level of exercise, these athletes often experience unhealthy weight gain which leads to many other negative health issues.

What Your Body Does with Food

The number shown on the scale as your weight at any given moment is the result of a basic formula:

$$\text{Calories Out} - \text{Calories In} = \text{Weight Change}$$

Here is the "conversation" that takes place in your body after eating a high-calorie meal and failing to expend that fuel:

Brain: Wow, with all this fuel, he must be preparing for something big. Stomach, get to processing.

Stomach: I'm on it. Give me about forty minutes and I'll have the energy ready to go.

Intestines (about 40 minutes later): Thanks for sending this fuel, but what am I supposed to do with it? It's not very good stuff. Hey, Brain, are you sure he's going to be physically active soon?

Brain: Why else would he eat so much?

Intestines: Well, he hasn't been active for years. I'm just going off experience here, but you're the smart one, so I'll go along with you.

Blood: Hey there, Intestines, what do you have for me today?

Intestines: It's not good, but Brain says he's going to use it quickly. Better get it out to all the muscle cells.

Blood: I'll do the best I can, but you know the walls in these vessels are getting clogged up because he hasn't exercised in years. I can only do so much with this junk. It's hard to move it around, so sometimes I just drop it off on the vessel walls because I can't carry it any longer.

Muscle Cells: Hey there, Blood, why are you waking me up? Go away.

Blood: Sorry, but Brain says this time is different. He's really going to do something physical this time. You better get ready.

Muscle Cells: You gonna fall for that one again? How many times has he said that? I know, I know; two weeks ago he thought he was Michael Jordan and tried to play pick-up ball with his kid's friends. Oh the horror!

Blood: Look, I know this junk is not the best for energy. You'll just have to make do.

Muscle Cells: *We are not going to process this junk just yet. If he doesn't do something physical soon, we'll just have Blood come pick it up and take it over to the Fat Cells. They'll store it for us.*

Blood: Hey Muscle Cells, I'm back to pick up your waste.

Muscle Cells: Sorry, Buddy, I didn't produce any energy from this junk. Take it over to the Fat Cells and have them store it. If he ever does decide to exercise, we'll use it then.

Blood: You got it, Buddy. I sure was hoping today would be the day because it's getting harder and harder to make it through these vessels. The pressure is almost more than I can take. If some regular exercise doesn't happen soon I may just blow up. Hey, Fat Cells…

Fat Cells: Gimme, gimme, gimme!

Blood: Settle down. Here's your junk. I'm sure you'll get more later today, too.

Fat Cells: We love it, *we love it*, WE LOVE IT! He cares for us. He feeds us. We are so loved.

Blood: Dudes, relax. You do realize you're killing us, right?

Fat Cells: No, it's just the opposite; we're the ones he's going to call on when he finally does that huge physical activity in the future.

Blood: Can you at least stop squishing all his organs?

Fat Cells: We can't help it. Hey, Brain, that last deposit was really salty. Do you think you could do us a favor and send down something sugary? And quickly!

Brain: Well, I know I shouldn't, but how about a soda? That will get to you the quickest.

Fat Cells: That would be great!

Granted, that is not a very scientific account of what happens during digestion. Here's a more accurate one: In your brain there are synapses firing all the time, even in your sleep. The transmission of neurons – the communication that occurs across these synapses – is what causes both conscious and subconscious thoughts and actions in your body. You do not have to think about breathing in order to breathe because these neurotransmissions are occurring constantly. Synapses are the initial step in the feeling of hunger. From there, like falling dominoes, the nerves instruct the different organs in the digestive system to prepare to work.

We are all trained to eat breakfast, lunch, and dinner at certain times of the day. Over time our brains become conditioned to signal hunger at those times of the day. If you are a parent, think of your kids before they were old enough for school. They seemed to want to eat all the time. Once kids begin school, the routine of the school day conditions them to eat a meal in the middle of the day, and their synapses fire to notify their stomachs to produce acid in order to begin digesting food at that time of day.

When food is digested it travels from the stomach through the small intestine and into the large intestine. During the trip, nutrients and minerals are extracted, primarily by the walls of the small intestine; absorbed into the bloodstream; and transported around the body.

Glucose is a simple sugar and a known source of energy for animals, including humans. It is commonly found in carbohydrates and foods that contain simple sugars. As food is broken down during the digestive process, glucose is absorbed into the bloodstream, providing the body with energy. Excess glucose is stored in the form of glycogen, which gets deposited in the fat cells if it is not used quickly. Poor-quality nutrients are also absorbed into the bloodstream. The issue then becomes where to deposit those nutrients, because the cells in your body do not want them. They either get deposited into the fat cells or, in the case of low-density lipoprotein cholesterol (LDL), cling to the sides of the blood vessels, increasing blood pressure and starting you down the path to heart disease.

Amino acids are high-quality nutrients that are commonly broken down from proteins in foods. They are critical to proper cell growth and structure and are the building blocks of muscle tissue, which means they play a vital role in burning fat.

The powerhouses inside each cell of the body are the organelles called mitochondria. They create energy from nutrients via cellular respiration. Keeping your mitochondria healthy and active results in healthy cells; which means healthy organs, muscles, and bones; which means a healthy body. When you have a healthy body you can function physically without issues. Oh yeah, this also gets you into the 30 percent minority of Americans who are healthy.

So how do you take care of your mitochondria? Provide your body with high-quality nutrients rich in amino acids, vitamins, and minerals; and exercise on a regular basis, which allows the mitochondria to create energy more efficiently, fortify the cell structure, and remove waste from the cells created by cellular respiration.

Food is meant to fuel your body from meal to meal. When you eat more than you need, your body stores it as fat for future use. If you never use it, does your body realize this and decide to stop storing it? Just the opposite. At the very core of the process your body is on autopilot; it continues to store excess energy for future use. As you age, the problem is not the amount of fat you have stored up but the effect that fat has on your internal organs.

It should be clear that the largest contributors to Americans' weight problems are poor diet and lack of exercise. But how did we get here? Our diet changed with the advent of fast food restaurants. I told myself when I started to write this book that it would not be a "bash fast food" book, but let's face the truth: fast food restaurants do not serve products with high nutritional value. Take the fast food hamburger, for instance. The calories in the signature hamburgers at the major chains range from 540 to 660. That's just the burger, and how often do you order the burger without a side and a drink? You better believe they are going to ask if you want fries with that – that's fast food 101. I'll discuss daily caloric needs in a later chapter, but let's assume for now that, as the government tells us, a 2,000-calorie diet is appropriate for all people. With just a single hamburger, without cheese, you have consumed one-fourth to one-third of your recommended daily calories.

Chemistry tells us that burning one pound of fat in a lab releases about 3,500 calories of energy. The mindset then becomes: burn an extra 3,500 calories and lose a pound of fat. In real life it takes more than that to lose a pound because your body constantly adapts to the fuel you give it and your physical activity. Your body first uses the energy created by your most recent meal before it begins to break down stored fat. But to keep the formula simple, let's just say that if you eat 2,000 calories of food a day, you need to burn 2,500 calories a day to burn off one pound of fat per week.

Using myself as an example, I completed a 3.2-mile run at a seven-minute-per-mile pace and burned 358 calories doing so. I'd have to do that about 10 times to burn one pound of fat through exercise alone. Granted, I'm at my healthy weight, so for me maintenance is the name of the game. But that gives you an idea of how the formula works.

Calories are one thing, but the bigger fast food issue is the sodium in the hamburgers. Most of them contain over half the daily sodium consumption limit established by the government. While most Americans will tell you that our major food problems are sugary and fatty foods, salt is the bigger problem. We are addicted to salt, and it is killing us. Add to your hamburger a large fries and a large soda – because, let's face it, you get more bang for your buck with a large over a medium – and you've exceeded half your daily caloric need, and almost hit the 2,300mg recommended *limit* of salt, before getting your free soda refill.

So what's the better choice at a fast food restaurant? The grilled chicken salad, right? It does have fewer calories than most of the other items on the menu, but the salt content can be even higher than that of the signature burger. The salad with fruit, nuts, and grilled chicken looks great from a caloric standpoint but has half the salt you should consume in a day – in just one dish.

Our addiction to salt is unnecessary and dangerous. We should not be adding any salt to our food – not while preparing it and not when it is served. I proved this point by not adding salt to my food for several years. Then in 2017 I had my annual physical, including a full blood workup. My blood sodium was 139 milliequivalents per liter, right in the middle of the normal range of 136 to 144. Granted, one test is a small sample size, but it proved to me that I do not need to eat excess salt to have enough in my body.

Why Is Salt So Bad?

We use salt as a seasoning and as a preserving compound. Salt has been used to preserve foods, particularly meats, since the time of the Old Testament. They did not have refrigerators and freezers as we do now. Salt kept their foods edible for a longer period of time. Fast-forward to today, and we still use salt for the same purpose. Almost every processed food contains salt to provide a longer shelf life. But we don't need to keep a bag of pasta for two years before we use it. And yes, there are processed products in your pantry that have a shelf life of two years or longer – check the packages yourself. With refrigeration in every home and grocery stores in every neighborhood, why would we need to store food for two years or longer?

Our food distribution system has taken convenience and bulk-volume discounting to a whole new level that is truly not necessary. But it is less expensive for manufacturers to produce mass quantities of products and add salt to preserve them so that they can produce food when they want to and not when you want it. Most Americans will tell you that preservative-free food is more expensive because it does not last as long on the shelf or in the refrigerator. While this is true when comparing the cost of a fresh item to that of a processed item, the overall cost of that extra salt to your health is not worth saving a few pennies.

We need to ingest fats to survive, but excess salt in our bodies attracts fat to it, thus we are preserving our insides through our addictions to salt and fats. Have you noticed that after eating a particularly salty evening meal you wake up the next morning feeling swollen, even to the point that your rings won't fit on your fingers? That's an immediate reaction to the excess salt. Your body is retaining fluid due to the salt. If you then eliminate salt from your diet for the next few days and drink water like you should, you will wind up in the bathroom a lot as your kidneys expel the excess fluid.

Sweat regulates your body temperature and removes toxins from your body. It's salty, and it's especially salty if you ingest excess salt. You might think that because you are losing salt in your sweat you must replace it, but your body is actually getting rid of excess salt because it's toxic to your overall health. You do not need to replace it. If you do you perpetuate a vicious cycle in which the excess salt in your body creates cravings for sugary foods such as carbohydrates.

Carbohydrates, or carbs, are a necessary part of a healthy diet. But salt-created cravings for carbs cause you to eat more foods that have high amounts of carbohydrates, which are typically also higher in salt. And the cycle continues, with pound after pound being preserved in your body.

Chances are high that when you get hungry and do not have a meal plan, you will fall prey to the "what is the closest thing to eat" solution due to these cravings, which also translates to "what is the fastest thing to eat." You will likely bypass even a healthy option that's already in your refrigerator for the fast-food option that looks so delicious in the advertisement.

What Is China Telling Us?

I've focused on Americans so far, but let's look at a really interesting thing happening in China. In the 1980s, when China was still pretty closed off to the ways of the Western world, just 7 percent of the population was overweight or obese. A very popular, very American fast food restaurant made its debut in China in 1990. The World Health Organization reported that as of 2016, 32.3 percent of China's population was overweight, and over 10 percent was obese. That is a pretty significant increase in just over 25 years. Statistics also show that in areas of higher population, the percentage of obese people is growing faster than in rural areas of China. Beijing, for instance, has an obesity rate of 25.9 percent, while the national average is 11.9 percent, not to mention those who are overweight but not obese. The introduction of American fast food has drastically and quickly changed the health of the Chinese people, and not for the better.

(https://www.theguardian.com/sustainable-business/2017/jan/09/obesity-fat-problem-chinese-cities and http://www.chinadaily.com.cn/china/2017-06/28/content_29921273.htm)

It's Time to Move On from the Past

I don't spend a lot of time dwelling on the past. I prefer to forgive, forget, and move on. I am like that with my clients as well. I don't judge them for how they got into the shape they're in; we address the issue and move forward to a solution. So let's look into the future for a moment. What if I could show you how to add 10 years to your life to enjoy in retirement? You would probably like that idea, right?

If you read Ben Tinker's CNN article cited earlier called "US Life Expectancy Drops for Second Year in a Row," you will find that male life expectancy in the US is at 76.1

years. (http://www.cnn.com/2017/12/21/health/us-life-expectancy-study/index.html) For an American man born in 1960 or later, the age to receive Social Security Retirement (if it is still there, but that is a whole other issue) is set at 67. Here is a short timeline for that man based on current statistics for retirement, nursing-home stays, and death:

> 67 years old: retire
> 74 years old: be admitted to a nursing home in which he
>   stays until death
> 76 years old: die
> (http://www.mylifesite.net/blog/post/so-ill-probably-
> need-long-term-care-but-for-how-long)

Statistics give him, at best, seven years of retirement. He will work his tail off for 45-plus years in the workforce in order to relax and enjoy seven years of retirement (at an age when it is difficult to enjoy physical activities if he has been overweight or obese for years). If he makes it to age 65 with a healthy body he can expect to live to 83. If he makes it to age 75 with a healthy body he can expect to live to 86. THAT IS 10 MORE YEARS than the predictions cited above!

A healthy body is one with a normal BMI (29.3 percent of the current male population) and no signs of chronic disease. (Health, United States, 2016, National Center for Health Statistics (Hyattsville, MD, 2017), table 15: "Life expectancy at birth, at age 65, and at age 75, by sex, race, and Hispanic origin: United States")

Now check out this amazing statistic: 31.3 percent of US males will make it to 86 years of age. Do you think it's a stretch to say that the 29.3 percent of males with a normal

BMI will be in that 31.3 percent? I think there's a pretty good chance these men will stay healthy. That means that of the 70 percent of overweight and obese males in the US today, 2 percent will make it to 86 years of age.

Which statistic do you want to fall into?

CHAPTER 2

WHAT'S WRONG WITH OUR DIET?

*Do not you know that your body is the temple of the Holy
Spirit, who lives in you and who was given to you by God?
You do not belong to yourselves but to God; he bought you
for a price. So use your bodies for God's glory.*

– 1 Corinthians 6:19-20

Remember the formula:

Calories Out – Calories In = Weight Change

We can all agree that this is a pretty simple formula, but
real life is rarely that simple. Why does it have to be so hard?
If we are honest with ourselves we would have to admit that
we made it this hard.

When Did *Diet* Become a Bad Word?

Okay, so *diet* is a four-letter word. But that is truly the
only similarity it has with the traditional four-letter profane
words in our lexicon. Here is the definition of *diet* from
Merriam-Webster:

1. a: food and drink regularly provided or consumed
   b: habitual nourishment
   c: the kind and amount of food prescribed for a person or animal for a special reason
   d: a regimen of eating and drinking sparingly so as to reduce one's weight

2. a: something provided or experienced repeatedly

Nowhere in the definition does it say "vulgar," which the dictionary does use to describe words traditionally considered profane. So by definition, *diet* is not a bad word. It simply describes what we eat and drink. But we have made the phrase "going on a diet" synonymous with getting a root canal, especially when we are compelled to go on a diet by medical professionals – those evil doctors and their desire for us to live long, healthy lives.

Going on a diet is not a bad thing. It can be difficult, yes. But it is an indication that a person cares about improving their health. And while that is a good thing in theory, it means change, and we don't like change.

That is the true issue – change. No matter what kind of change is contemplated, even pocket change, we typically do not respond well to the idea of change. I address how to embrace change in the next chapter, but before we can get to the solution we have to know what the problem is.

My high school chemistry teacher was Brother Malcolm Melcher. When a student gave an answer to an equation without properly defining it, Brother Malcolm would jump in and ask, for example, "Nine point four what? Horses, cars, pencils?" While he was not the teacher to pull jokes on, or to answer incorrectly on purpose to evoke a reaction from, we all thought it was hilarious.

That story illustrates that a solution cannot solve a problem if it does not fully state the result; and you cannot fully state the result if you do not understand the problem. So what is the problem with your diet?

Is Advertising Killing You?

Are you living paycheck to paycheck in regard to your health? In other words, is "When is the next meal?" the only thought you have in regard to your health? I believe a vast majority of people in America live this way. We drive to work, at lunch time, and back home, waiting for a restaurant sign to grab our attention. Why do you think they make signs that rotate with lights and fancy graphics to advertise the daily specials? Those restaurant owners know they must stand out in the crowd to get your attention. They know that you operate without a solid plan. They know you better than you know yourself.

Plan your meals ahead of time in order to avoid the temptations of harmful foods, just as you have a budget in place to avoid impulse spending. Otherwise the immediacy of the unplanned hunger attack will take over and you will fall prey to fast-food and junk-food advertising. It is amazing to me how similar a health budget and a financial budget are. Each is extremely important if you are going to be successful in that respective area. But what marketing professionals know is that most Americans have neither kind of budget or plan. That's why there are so many advertisements for mass-produced items and far fewer for high-end items. Take the automotive industry. Chevrolet, Dodge, Ford, etc. constantly run TV ads because they know that low- and middle-income folks watch a lot of TV. They know where to find you. Auto dealers also know they are competing for that one dollar you are trying to save. But luxury lines like Ferrari, Lamborghini, Bentley, etc. don't need to advertise because they have built their brands as status symbols. If you want the best, you know where to go. It is highly unlikely that you can buy a Bentley for the cost of a Chevy unless it's 25 years old and has 250,000 miles on it and the upholstery is ruined. You get what you pay for.

Now apply that principle to your health. It's the fast-food and quick-dining joints that are advertised the most. Not all of the food served at these restaurants is bad for your health, but you have to question how a meal from a dollar menu can contain the same nutrition as a high-quality home-cooked meal. That dollar has to cover the cost of so much overhead that you know that dollar item has to contain the cheapest ingredients.

Let's consider a hamburger on the dollar menu. There is a bun, a meat patty, condiments, and possibly lettuce, tomato, onion, and/or pickles that have to be paid for. Then there is the cost of the labor to cook the burger, the labor to take your money, the packaging, the maintenance of the cooking equipment, managers who have to be paid, a building to be paid for, taxes to be paid – I could keep going.... Oh, and there should be profit, but they make their profit on the fountain drinks. Nowhere else does a fountain drink cost an average of $2.00. You are not getting anywhere near the value for a fountain drink there – especially because the cup is filled with ice first, unless of course you stay at the restaurant all day and get dozens of refills. Compare that price to a 12-pack of 12-ounce sodas that sells for $4.50 at your grocery store.

But don't go out and buy a 12-pack of soda because it's the better financial deal; it's still a horrible choice for your health. There are roughly 150 calories and 40 grams of sugar in a typical 12-ounce soft drink. In most cases that sugar is in some highly processed form because very few manufacturers use pure cane sugar due to its cost. All the major soft drink companies spend millions if not billions a year on advertising to get you to drink their brand. And it works. Even with all the research and publicity about how bad soft drinks are for you, they are still the most common drink ordered in restaurants. There's also a little bit of sodium in each of these drinks as well; that's why they have such a long shelf life.

If you think you're better off because you drink diet soda, that's not exactly correct. Sure diet drinks might have zero calories, but they are processed even further than regular soft drinks in order to remove the calories. Then they add artificial sweeteners back in. There is preliminary research that shows a link between artificial sweeteners and cancer. (https://www.mdanderson.org/publications/focused-on-health/october-2014/does-diet-soda-cause-cancer.html) There is no nutritional value in either regular or diet soda, and they increase your cravings for sugars and salts. Also mentioned in the article cited above is that studies showed that diet drinks actually led to a higher level of obesity due to the body's inability to properly metabolize the unnatural ingredients. Another danger is the carbonation. Studies showed that carbonation had a negative effect on people with lung disease. (https://www.livestrong.com/article/550595-effects-of-carbonated-drinks-on-lungs) And

I believe that our lungs do not function at prime efficiency when carbonation is present in the body, because if it's not good for unhealthy lungs, why would it be good for healthy lungs? Perhaps those lungs became unhealthy due in part to constant exposure to carbonation. I'm not a pulmonologist, but as I mentioned in the introduction, I have twice had a spontaneous pneumothorax, and as a result I have become more aware of lung research. Filtered water, my drink of choice, has no calories, hydrates you properly, and does not lead to cravings.

Don't Restaurants Care about Our Health?

Before you go down the conspiracy theory route, remember that all for-profit restaurants have one major goal they want to achieve: *profits*. There are some that care about their customers' health but very few will go out of business to keep you healthy. So it comes back down to – you get what you pay for.

There is another old adage that I like to remind people of when it comes to food: You are what you eat. When you eat meals made from ingredients that have poor nutritional value, your body ends up with poor nutritional value. God made us as pretty remarkable beings, but our cells can only do so much. A lot of people unfortunately think of their bodies as similar to water filters – whatever they put in is going to come out clean and useful. But we aren't filtering our food for use by someone else, like a water filter does; we are digesting it to fuel our bodies.

Instead of a filter, think of your body as the engine that it is. The most obvious analogy is the different types of automotive fuel. There are three typical choices: regular, premium, and super. Fuel companies advertise that if you want high performance from your vehicle you should use super; that the better grade (or quality) fuel provides better performance. Seems obvious, right? We are all aware that a high-performing vehicle is desirable. But in most cases there is very little difference between the types of unleaded fuel, and people choose their fuel based on what they can afford, knowing that using the regular could lead to performance issues and a trip to the mechanic a little sooner than later. It's a risk most people are willing to take. I take that risk as well, but I also have a great mechanic who is honest and treats me fairly. The worst-case scenario is that the vehicle will break down and not be repairable, at which point you simply sell it for what you can and buy another one.

It's a little more difficult to do that with your body. Sure, there are cutting-edge medical procedures that can do wondrous things to correct your mistakes. Those come with a price – a financial price but also a physical price. If you have never had surgery, I can tell you that recovery from any surgery is frustratingly slow. You lose stamina and strength while you are in the hospital. Whether you get therapy after your surgery or not, it's an uphill climb to get back to normal physically. Recovery takes an emotional toll on you as well.

Eating nutritionally poor food and refusing to make exercise a habit will cause health issues, guaranteed. While it's not impossible to recover from some of the health issues of these choices – obesity, heart disease, chronic illnesses, diabetes, etc. – you can't very well trade yourself in for a newer model. Once the damage has been done, reversing it can be a slow and painful process.

I'm a Picky Eater and I Hate Vegetables

My gut reaction when someone tells me they are a picky eater is to laugh. Do you know how silly that sounds? In reality, we are all picky eaters. We all pick what we eat. Have you ever heard a vegetarian or vegan announce themselves as a picky eater? No; they're proud of their ability to choose wisely what they want to eat. When someone says they don't like healthy food, they are really saying, "I am not going to eat healthy food because I am not used to it."

The real issue is that you are a *trained* eater. You have been trained by your parents or you trained yourself to eat only certain foods. Foods high in processed sugar, salt, saturated and trans fats, and high fructose corn syrup create cravings for more foods of the same type, which is how the cycle begins.

As mentioned in the previous chapter, salt drives cravings for sweets and carbs. Eating these sugars causes chemical reactions in your body that eventually create an excess of serotonin, a neurotransmitter, in the brain. Among other things, serotonin improves your mood. This does two things: increases the release of dopamine in the brain, and trains you to connect that food type to happiness. (https://www.livestrong.com/article/96983-causes-sugar-cravings)

Dopamine is a neurotransmitter associated with causing addictions. Ever wonder why common street drugs are called "dope"? It's because they cause a release of dopamine, which is responsible for addictive behavior. High levels of dopamine have been recorded in athletes after exercise, gamblers after a big score, and drug users.

The cool thing about dopamine is that you can use it to your advantage. Exercising releases dopamine naturally because God designed your body to move. (So start exercising!) When you start to eat healthier foods, think to yourself how happy you are to be eating healthy; how great your body will feel after eating quality foods meal after meal. These positive affirmations release dopamine into your system, eventually changing the way your brain relates to healthy foods. You get a happiness feeling from eating a carrot, an apple, or another healthy snack, so you no longer need that chocolate bar to feel happy. You're training yourself to connect healthy foods to happiness. (https://www.livestrong.com/article/356769-supplements-to-help-build-dopamine-serotonin)

You are not picky in the least. You are trained. As an adult responsible for your own food, you make a choice to eat healthy or not to eat healthy. Once you realize it's a choice and that you're not chained to your conditioning, you can break the cycle. But it takes time to do this, which is one reason people have such a hard time sticking to diets.

Time... Where Is the Time?

We live in a fast-paced world. Our lives are moving so fast we have almost forgotten to live them. We have spouses, kids, pets, family and friends, businesses to run, volunteering to do, religious commitments, community obligations – where is the time to invest in a healthy lifestyle? In fact, I'm writing this at 2:27am because this is when I have the time. And I'm not a night owl. I'm usually asleep by 9:30 because I'm up at 5:00 starting my work day.

I'm sure you have heard the saying "Time is money." I think we have forgotten that we need to spend some of that time on our health. Yes, it takes time to cook a meal at home versus picking it up at the local drive-thru. Yes, it takes time to plan healthy meals for the week. Yes, it takes time to shop for groceries and spend time evaluating which products are healthy. Yes, it takes time to plan for a proper exercise routine each week. I totally understand that your time is valuable and you don't feel you have enough to spend it on your health. But if you don't take the time now, you will not have the time later when you want to play after you retire.

Money... I Don't Have the Money!

I hear it all the time: "It costs too much to eat healthy." That's just baloney. (But don't go out and buy bologna – seriously not good for you!) Yes, healthy foods themselves cost more than what you were trained to eat, but only if you compare the straight food costs. When you add in all the other costs associated with an unhealthy lifestyle you find that eating healthy is far less expensive.

Here are a few of the hidden costs you pay by eating unhealthy foods:

- Higher health insurance rates
- Higher out-of-pocket medical expenditures
- Increased need for prescription medication
- Lower productivity at work
- More frequent sick days and time lost at work
- Higher life insurance rates

A hidden gem of eating healthy is that you learn to eat less. When you eat less of foods that are a little more expensive, your overall food budget is at least the same and in most cases far lower than if you overeat less expensive foods, especially because you're likely to eat at home rather than constantly invest in the overhead at your local fast food joint.

Mom Always Said I'm Big-Boned

I'm sorry about what your mom told you, but you are not big-boned. Do some people have different skeletal frames? Absolutely. But the size of your body frame has nothing to do with your fat retention or your poor food choices. What your mom said is what's driving your food choices, reinforcing that you will be large your whole life.

Your perception of yourself might have more to do with your food choices than you are willing to admit. "Might as well eat what I want because I am genetically disadvantaged." This defeatist thinking prevents you from living a healthy lifestyle. Change your mindset in this regard, and a healthy lifestyle is entirely achievable.

I Have Bad Genes

A lot of people think they cannot lose weight and get in shape because they have bad genes. Of course, genes are not bad – your body was just trained incorrectly. Yes, some people have faster metabolisms than others. The cool thing is you can control your metabolism.

A lot of the people who were on the popular TV show *The Biggest Loser* came from families with histories of obesity and weight issues, yet they lost weight. They reached their ideal body weight because they ate healthy and exercised. What you saw on the show was just a glimpse into their week. It did not show that those contestants were exercising eight hours,

10 hours, 12 hours a day into their target-heart-rate range. So of course they were burning fat like crazy and could lose 12, 15, or 30 pounds a week. Most of us do not have eight to 12 hours a day to dedicate to exercise, so it's not likely you will lose 12 to 30 pounds a week. It is widely agreed in the medical community that a healthy way to lose weight is at a rate of one or two pounds a week. You can do that easily by getting into your target-heart-rate range for 30 minutes a day, three to five days a week. Combine that with a healthy diet, and you will easily burn one or two pounds of fat per week.

CHAPTER 3

SIMPLE SOLUTION?

Do not be wise in your own eyes; fear the LORD and shun evil. This will bring health to your body and nourishment to your bones.

– Proverbs 3:7-8

It's a simple formula, right? This is all you need to know to lose weight:

Calories Out – Calories In = Weight Change

So why would I write another word in this book? Because. It. Is. Just. Not. That. Easy.

So What Is the Solution?

The solution is not counting calories or reading nutrition labels. It is not going vegetarian or vegan or stockpiling supplements. It is not trying to find the perfect balance of carbohydrates, protein, and fiber. Those are tactics that can be used to arrive at a healthy lifestyle, but the real solution is *you!* You have to change.

Simple, right? But just as I would caution someone who is betrothed that they should not assume they will be able to change their future spouse, changing yourself is even more difficult. (Be there to support your partner as they seek change, but do not try to force it on them; it's a good way to end up sleeping on the couch.)

Dave Ramsey, a nationally known financial counselor and author, often states that people do not change their financial habits until "they get sick and tired of being sick and tired." His point is that you will not change until a catalyst acts on you. In the world of finance, that could be when you realize the debt game just does not work. Or the catalyst could be bankruptcy, foreclosure, or large medical bills.

What Is Your Catalyst?

Just as with your finances, you have a choice regarding your health. You can choose to continue to live an unhealthy lifestyle until a catalyst acts on you in the form of a catastrophic illness. This is where your health and finances collide. Extreme illness, disease, and surgeries are expensive and can cripple most families financially and emotionally.

Again it comes back to *you*. You have the choice to be the catalyst to change your ways. I highly recommend this option. Take control of your health. Act against the restaurants clamoring for your every dollar. Embrace that the food you eat is truly fuel for your body. Do you want your body to be a Ferrari or a Yugo? No matter what your other life circumstances, you control what your body looks like and how it operates.

A high school friend of mine got a brand new Mustang as his first car, but did not know he had to change the oil. Several months later he blew the engine because he had not been caring for his car properly. That bypass surgery catalyst in your future will amount to the same thing – blowing your engine.

The Importance of Healthy Meal Plans

Having a plan for your meals is a step in the right direction, but making sure it is a healthy plan is key. Planning to eat food low in nutritional value is not a good plan. That's like saying your plan to get rich is to rob a few banks; you might get away with it once or twice, but eventually you are going to be caught and spend some time in jail with no freedoms. Eating is similar in that we all want the freedom to eat whatever we want to whenever we want to, but eventually the health police – that is, your body – is going to tell you that you can no longer eat like that without drastic repercussions in your life – like disease and death.

The goal of a healthy meal plan is to eat foods high in nutritional value in the proper portions at the proper time of day. As Stephen Covey stated, "Begin with the end in mind." Knowing what a healthy meal plan looks like is critical to reaching the goal of a healthy lifestyle.

What typically derails people is not that there is a shortage of information about how to create a healthy meal plan, but which information applies best to them. There are even programs that provide you with all the food you need in prepackaged meals. There are plans that have you count calories. The government has published diet recommendations for the American public for many decades.

The way I create a meal plan is to first consider my client's current eating habits. I address the worst mistakes such as soft drinks, processed foods, and portion sizes. But each person is different. A husband and wife might have equally poor BMIs, but their nutritional needs are different. Differences in gender, height, weight, and age dictate different approaches to meal plans. This does not mean that you will forever be cooking two different meals. Your meals will generally be the same as those for the other people you eat with, but the portion sizes will be different. Healthy food is good for you at any age; it's the portion sizes that change. That's as simple as the obvious difference in portions for children and adults.

I look at meal plans from the perspective of transforming your brain. If you can train your brain to crave healthy foods in the proper portions (which is entirely possible), you will not need to worry about counting calories, protein, fiber, or any other nutrients. Proper portions of healthy foods will provide you with all the nutrition you need. With the proper nutrients in your system, the exercise you do will flush out toxins and actually create cravings for healthy foods. Ever wonder why your healthy coworker can enjoy a carrot or apple as an afternoon snack? It's because their brain and cells understand the high-quality nutrients they are receiving.

Following a healthy meal plan for one week does not result in a lifestyle. If it were that easy – well, it would be that easy. As you age, your nutritional needs change. As you exercise more, your nutritional needs change. As your body composition changes (your proportion of fat to muscle), your nutritional needs change. So it's not as simple as eating 1,500 calories a day. People tend to yo-yo diet, losing weight only to gain it back months later, because what they need to eat when they weigh 200 pounds and are trying to lose 50 pounds is not the same as what they need to eat when they reach 150 pounds and are trying to maintain that level. Not making that transition in a healthy way leads to giving up on their plan and going back to unhealthy eating habits.

Earlier I described how the synapses work in your brain. The key to a healthy lifestyle is to provide your body with the nutrients necessary to create the enzymes and chemicals that your cells depend on to function in the way God created them to. God designed you to be healthy, but to honor that design you have to take control of what goes in your mouth.

Fighting Your Conditioning

Being the catalyst that changes your diet to a healthy diet is both a mental task and an emotional task. This is not where I tell you that weight loss is all mental – count your calories and you will be fine; just the opposite: Don't get bogged down in counting calories and grams of this and that. Most of us find out pretty early in school if we enjoy that kind of detailed math. No offense if you're a math nerd, but most of us don't enjoy it and don't have the time for it even if we do. So why do it with something as important as your health?

The mental task is to tell yourself to stick to your plan throughout the day, especially when you first embark on your meal plan. If you don't consistently defend your plan to yourself in your mind you will fall prey to the nearest advertisement, restaurant sign, or sound of soda fizz. Your subconscious has been programmed by your poor eating habits to override your body's nutritional needs, so you have to outmaneuver your subconscious thinking.

In every area of life – health, finances, work, relationships, etc. – *needs versus wants* is a struggle. Think about an area of your life in which you're successful – everything is great in that area right now. I bet you are happy about that area because all of your needs in that area are being met. Now look at an area in which you're not doing so well. Is it because you're going after your wants without having first satisfied your needs in that area?

It's easy to see that the majority of Americans are eating what they want to eat before satisfying their nutritional needs. If you meet all your nutritional needs first, not only does your health improve but you stop craving junk food. That is how you end the cycle. If you want the data about whether or not you are meeting your nutritional needs, have a comprehensive blood test done. If any levels are not within normal limits, you are suffering nutritionally.

Most Americans have been brought up thinking that junk food is a reward, from being given a candy bar for being good in the grocery store to being served a special dessert for good grades. As a society we have put undue stress on our health by tying food to emotions. My kids are different from "normal" kids because while they enjoy splurging, they routinely pass up sweets for fruit. Yes, they love ice cream, but they do not request it or crave it every night because we serve it only on occasion and don't identify it as a reward.

I don't mean to dismiss the emotional effect food has on our brains. It has been proven scientifically that foods do,

Simple Solution?

in fact, stimulate the pleasure areas of our brains. But we have expanded that effect far beyond what God intended. In extreme cases we have pushed the role of junk food to one of companionship. We often seek out food in times of stress or depression. This is when to employ the mental process to work with the emotional one.

Mental and Emotional Teamwork

One of the biggest challenges in our society is learning how to communicate and deal with our emotions in a positive manner. Many of us eat in accordance with our emotions. We "eat" our family issues, work issues, health issues, and anything that causes unexpected stress. When we know the stress is coming we can prepare for it; it's those unexpected stressors that result in emotional eating. An example commonly portrayed in television shows and movies is a woman being dumped by her boyfriend and opting to stay at home alone and eat a carton of ice cream. The next day she recounts her evening to a friend and is now upset not only about the former boyfriend but also about binge-eating a half-gallon of ice cream.

To overcome the habit of emotional eating you have to be on guard and ready to act at any moment – the "mental task" part. You must be mentally prepared at all times. The best way to succeed at this mental task is to create a sound plan, become familiar with your plan, work your plan, and live your plan. Without a plan, your subconscious takes over. In today's digital age, information comes at us at lightning speed. Our emotions can change in an instant, which means our habit of eating emotionally, especially junk food, can pop up at any time.

I'm sure you have heard the saying "No one ever plans to fail; they fail to plan." It's very true in regard to how you deal with your emotions. Without a solid support system – your plan – you will turn to food to deal with your emotions without even realizing you are doing it.

Why are you ready for a nap in the middle of the afternoon? It has everything to do with how you fueled your body at lunch – or rather *improperly* fueled it. Did you act on a sound plan for your health and eat for the tasks of the day, or did you eat based on your emotions and the stress of the morning, thus setting yourself up for an energy deficit during the afternoon? If you eat a healthy breakfast, followed by a light mid-morning snack, and then a healthy lunch, you will not have a mid-afternoon sugar crash because your body is not riding a sugar roller coaster. I recommend an afternoon snack as well, but not because a mid-afternoon energy crash is normal. Your body needs nutrients throughout the day. When you don't provide them at regular intervals (more often than the typical three meals a day) you become susceptible to the sugar roller coaster. The purpose of regular snacks is to keep your body's sugar level as even as possible, avoiding extreme highs and extreme lows.

Why do you think we have happy hour? After a particularly hard day at work, would you rather go home and deal with the stress in a difficult but healthy way, or forget about it by drinking and eating it away? You are basically choosing between exercising and drinking/eating snack foods. It's especially easy to fall into the happy-hour trap if you're single. Not that hanging with coworkers after a difficult day at work is a bad thing, but the poor nutritional decisions typically made during a happy-hour gathering are the trap.

Having a plan that incorporates both your mental awareness and your emotional stability is key. Knowing your meal plan, knowing the healthy options, and knowing your reasons for being strong-willed enough to stick to it lead to the emotional stability you need to achieve the healthy lifestyle you crave.

Exercising is a great way to stabilize your emotions. It relieves stress, which is usually a large contributor to your emotional state. Another great way to stabilize your emotions is to share your feelings with someone. If you're married, your spouse is probably your first choice. But it can be a close friend, your pastor, another family member, or the very person who sent your emotions into a tailspin. Communicating your emotions validates your stance and relieves your stress, especially if you are emotionally charged to the point of tears. Crying when communicating your emotions is a built-in soul-cleansing faculty that God gave you. After this conversation (and potential cry) you can move past the stressful issue without the urge to eat your feelings away.

The Role of Accountability

Can you do it on your own? Most of us can't. You revert to your old ways at the first sign of difficulty – unless, of course, some major medical catalyst happened to you that precludes giving up. Often the thought of going through such a trauma again is enough to hold anyone accountable to themselves for their new healthy lifestyle.

You want to prevent that medical catalyst and take control of your life by being your own catalyst. That is hard enough that I recommend finding someone who will hold you accountable to your new lifestyle, whether it's your spouse, a family member, a friend, a coach, or a trainer. It can even be a group like a Weight Watchers group. When you start out you need that support so you won't get sidetracked.

There is always something special going on to tempt you with sweets or a big, unhealthy meal. You will have to let the people in your life know what you're doing so they can support you or at least not undermine your efforts when you're faced with holiday and family gatherings. Even better, find someone to do the plan with you.

Accountability is no longer as esteemed in our society as it used to be. So many now want to do it on their own.

Be all you can be!

Just do it!

You got this!

Make it happen.

Shock everyone.

All those slogans don't really tell the truth: You are most productive when you lean on the advice of others, when others support you, and when others hold you accountable. That is when success happens.

Don't make achieving a healthy lifestyle harder than it needs to be. Don't put so much pressure on yourself that you never start. Taking the first step is difficult, but by taking just one simple first step you can be on your way. Staying on the path before it becomes habit, before it becomes real, before it becomes a lifestyle, is difficult too, but with an accountability partner you can see it through.

Skin in the Game

My friend keeps telling me that someday he will sign up for one of my programs because he knows he can be and needs to be in better health. We communicate every few weeks or so on social media and talk on the phone about every two or three months. I have come straight out and offered him a package I think would be good for him, but he wasn't ready. He said he needed to get in a little better condition on his own first before he would be ready. It's been about a year since that conversation and he's still in the same condition, although he keeps saying "one day... one day." I know you have to be emotionally ready to work on your health, and I wrote this book to help you see that today needs to be that day.

My first paying client has not yet achieved her goal, but she has made great strides. During our first phone call she was very timid, shy, and scared as we discussed her current health. She was grossly obese; in fact one of her biggest issues was that she was unable to walk very far without having to sit down due to her weight. This even affected her ability to perform her duties at work.

I did not speak to her again for about three months because I provided everything she needed via text and email. When we spoke again it was because she had sent an email that she was concerned I might misinterpret. As we talked on the phone I remember thinking, "Who is this person?" She was not the same person I had spoken with three months earlier. She was confident. She laughed. She was ready for the next challenge. This was 100 percent the result of exercise improving her self-esteem.

Contrast that to a very different result on the part of an acquaintance of mine I attempted to help. The first mistake I made was to make the first move versus his coming to me. While he was well aware that his current health status was poor, it was me who wanted him to do something about it. I gave him my services at no charge, which was the second mistake I made. Not only did he not truly want my help, now he did not even have to pay for it. I had removed the motivation of getting what he paid for.

To follow through on your goals you need to have some skin in the game, and financial skin is one of the most motivating kinds. No one wants to spend money on something and not get any results from it. So whether you pay a coach like me or put money aside to be used as a reward once you reach your goal, seeing money leave your hand can be a huge motivator to continue towards your goal and get results.

The Role of Coaching

It's easy to see why teams need coaches: everyone has to commit equally to the effort or the team concept doesn't work, and it's the coach's responsibility to ensure that happens. In individual sports such as tennis, golf, boxing, and track, you might think that being the greatest in the world is enough, but you still need a coach. Even though you might have more knowledge of the sport and more athletic ability than your coach, it's essentially impossible to maintain your level of achievement without a coach.

Roger Federer has had several coaches throughout his tennis career. Phil Mickelson has had several different swing coaches during his golf career. Muhammed Ali had several coaches who specialized in different aspects of boxing and fitness. Sprinter Usain Bolt had a coach; it might sound odd because all he had to do is run fast, but there is far more to it. Every great athlete needs someone to advise them, support them, and push them to the next level. Coaches can see when a foot placement is wrong or an arm angle is off, but coaching is far more than just the physical coaching of the sport. Coaches are also counselors and psychologists. Some athletes even hire a separate sport psychologist to help them reach their goals.

Golf might be the best sport to correlate with a healthy lifestyle. With track it's all about running, jumping, or throwing better than your competitor, but the stadium is always the same shape; the race is the same distance; the height to jump is the same for everyone. In boxing, the ring is the same size every time and you have just one other person to beat in the same amount of time in each boxing match. Tennis gets a little closer to the struggles of a healthy lifestyle because while the type of court surface can change, which affects the spin of the ball, all other circumstances of a tennis match are the same from match to match. Golf, though, is a whole different game each time you play. Golfers compete against each other, the weather, *and* the course. In a four-day tournament, the course even changes from day to day; placement on the tee boxes change; the locations of the holes on the greens change; each golfer's psyche changes from day to day based on how they are doing compared to their competitors. A golfer rarely hits the same exact shot twice, so they must trust their knowledge and abilities. What else does a professional golfer have to create an advantage? Their caddie – someone who helps with their psyche and motivation and provides input and feedback regarding shot selection as the competition unfolds.

This is very similar to a healthy lifestyle. If you think of your normal daily routine as an 18-hole golf course, the analogy holds in that the day never unfolds exactly as the day before it. You might have the same tasks two days in a row but rarely does the result match exactly. A coach will help you understand what to eat when, just as a golf coach teaches when to use a driver versus a putter. A coach can act as your caddie to address unexpected challenges to your healthy lifestyle, such as when your coworker brings you an entire cake for your birthday.

My client Trudy (not her real name) experienced this. I received a text message with a picture of a cake sitting on her desk. Her coworker did not know she was a month into a healthy lifestyle change. Trudy's question was "What do I do?" She was torn because she did not want to hurt her coworker's feelings but she knew this cake was not going to be good for her new lifestyle. A small piece of cake is not going to derail your entire plan, but an entire cake for a single person who has no one at home to share it with can easily derail a month's worth of work towards health.

Trudy had never told someone "No thank you" for a food gift before, primarily because she had never had a plan for her food before. I helped her process how to emotionally overcome the gift, and, finally believing in herself, she took the cake to her coworker and politely declined it. She told her coworker that she was on a new healthy lifestyle plan and the cake would not be good for her. She offered the compromise of placing the cake in the breakroom for the entire office to share. The coworker thought that was a great idea and complimented her on her new lifestyle. This did wonders for Trudy's self-esteem. She wasn't even tempted to eat a piece of the cake. (Tap in to this example when faced with something like it!)

Numbers for the Formula

I gave you a formula based on calories but then revealed the solution as an abstract *you*. Let me explain why numbers by themselves do not work.

A 2,000-calorie-per-day diet is widely characterized as a recommended diet. But as with everything in life, you have to look at the entire recommendation. That 2,000-calorie-per-day diet is for maintaining weight, for a certain gender, for someone of a certain height and weight, when exercising at a moderate to vigorous intensity level for an average of three hours a week.

Take someone like me, for an example – a male in my early forties, 5 foot 9 inches tall. If I exercise at a moderate level three to five times per week, I need to consume roughly 2,500 calories a day to maintain a weight of 150 pounds. But if I weighed 200 pounds, a 2,500-calorie-per-day diet would allow me to lose about one pound a week with that same level of exercise, and a 2,000-calorie-per-day diet would barely be enough to live on.

The term *daily caloric need* (DCN) refers to the number of calories you need each day to maintain your weight, accounting for how much you exercise. You can find a DCN calculator on my website, www.allinhealthandwellness.com. Play around with the formulas in the calculator. Plug in your numbers and see what it tells you. Then plug in your goal weight and see what you get. Use your spouse's numbers to see the difference that gender makes. *Basal metabolic rate* (BMR) is the number of calories you need to maintain your current weight without exercise – no energy output. That is simply what you need to stay alive.

So if DCN is what you need to maintain your current weight including moderate to high-intensity exercise, and BMR is what you need to maintain your weight without exercise, it should stand to reason that if you eat less than your DCN or BMR you will lose weight. Not exactly.

God created us with this other function called starvation mode. If you withhold calories to the point that your body thinks it is in starvation mode, you will not initially lose weight, and you can actually gain weight. Your body is trying to survive at all costs. It will stay in this mode for some time before eventually kicking into fat burning. But this is a very dangerous way to go about losing weight. Your brain gets used to surviving on very few nutrients from food, and without your brain telling you to eat more, your bodily systems start to work inefficiently. This type of weight-loss plan all too often leads to anorexia. That is not a disorder you want in your life.

With exercise, your DCN increases. Weight loss happens in a healthy way when you ingest fewer calories than your DCN and more than your BMR, coupled with moderate exercise. Yes, you can see greater weight loss if you ingest fewer calories than your BMR, but it is dangerous, as described above, and you greatly increase your risk of injury during exercise.

I don't want you to get caught up in the numbers, though. It can be very difficult to try to figure out exactly how many calories are in each meal, how many grams of protein, how many grams of fiber, how many carbohydrates, etc., etc., etc., starting on the first day of a diet. And a healthy meal plan does not require that you take in the same nutrition each day; the calorie count fluctuates from day to day based on your overall health goal and your exercise routine. Try to figure out your exact caloric intake and you will give up before you make it to 3:00pm on the first day – you will find yourself at the drive-thru of the nearest fast food restaurant ordering "the usual."

With a sound, healthy meal plan you do not have to think about the numbers. It will retrain your brain to eat the right numbers naturally. It will teach your body to crave the high-quality nutrients it needs.

As James R. Sherman wrote (often mistakenly attributed to C. S. Lewis), "You can't go back and make a new start, but you can start right now and make a brand new ending." Don't get depressed about the unhealthy life you have lived to this point; that will not help you succeed. Plant yourself in front of a mirror, stand tall, lift your head up, look straight into your eyes, and say this out loud:

I will be healthy for me. I am strong enough to fight off food temptations. I will not listen to others who do not support me. I will get help to navigate eating and exercise. I will mess up but I will not give up. I am not a failure. I can eat healthy foods. I can exercise. I do not fear change. I will be healthy!

CHAPTER 4

DEFINING A HEALTHY LIFESTYLE

*Dear friend, I pray that you may enjoy good health
and that all may go well with you, even as your soul is
getting along well.*

– 3 John 1:2

There is a lot of talk about the need to live a healthy lifestyle. Every person I come in contact with shares that they know they need to exercise and eat a healthy diet. So the problem is not that we don't know that a healthy lifestyle is important; it's that we don't really know what a healthy lifestyle is.

The Definition of a Healthy Lifestyle

A research study published in *Mayo Clinic Proceedings* in 2016 looked at characteristics of a healthy lifestyle and their association with cardiovascular disease. Let's look at the four indicators they used to define a healthy lifestyle:

- Exercise: 2.5 hours of moderate to high-intensity exercise per week

- Diet: Follow the government's nutritional recommendations

- Body composition: Have a body-fat percentage between 5 and 20 percent for men and 8 and 30 percent for women

- Smoking status: Be a non-smoker

The researchers studied approximately 5,000 people over a two-and-a-half-year period. They found that only 2.7 percent of study participants met all four indicators. (https://inbodyusa. com/blogs/inbodyblog/94523969-what-the-only-2-7-of-americans-live-healthy-lifestyles-study-says-about-body-fat) No wonder 70 percent of Americans are overweight or obese. Their findings could be skewed based on their participant pool. I don't know if they sought out a true cross-cultural sample or if they requested participants who were already overweight or obese, but even if they studied 5,000 overweight people, to find that only 2.7 percent were even attempting to live a healthy lifestyle is a staggeringly low number.

A healthy lifestyle is much more than eating healthy and exercising. A healthy lifestyle is a way of life. It is living life to the fullest with a healthy body, mind, and spirit. A healthy lifestyle is achieved through eating a healthy diet, maintaining a regular exercise routine, refraining from unhealthy habits such as smoking, connecting with those around you, and seeking wisdom from God.

The Difference between Healthy Living and Weight Loss

Going on a diet to lose weight does not automatically mean you are living a healthy lifestyle. On the flip side, losing weight is not necessarily a side effect of a healthy lifestyle. And not all weight-loss diets are healthy. This is one reason diets come and go as fads. Someone creates a diet plan; it works for some of their friends and clients; they begin to market it to the public; and eventually researchers study the diet to determine whether or not it is truly a healthy way to live. Some make the cut and some do not.

There are lots of ways to lose weight. Some are sold as shortcuts to your dream body. Some will work for you but not for your spouse. Too many people reject the tried and true formula I provided earlier for the quick fix. Some quick-fix diets work temporarily, but do not result in a healthy lifestyle. I know you have heard this statement from someone before: "I tried that diet. As soon as I got off it I gained all the weight back, plus more."

Quick fixes in any part of life are rarely good for you in the long run. Take winning the lottery. It is estimated that 70 percent of all lottery winners are broke again within seven years. (http://www.cleveland.com/business/index. ssf/2016/01/why_do_70_percent_of_lottery_w.html) If you have never lived with an abundance of money it is difficult to know how to act when you receive a windfall. It's easy to see how a lottery winner who does not seek financial counseling could blow through their winnings before even realizing what happened.

Another interesting statistic that correlates to health and finances is workplace engagement. How engaged you are in your work has a definite effect on how happy you are, primarily because you can avoid typical stressors when you are happy to be doing your work.

According to Gallup Poll's 2013 "State of the American Workplace" survey, American workers were growing more disengaged from their work. The poll discovered that of the approximately 100 million people in America who held full-time jobs, 30 percent were engaged and inspired at work. Fifty percent were disengaged, or what Gallup described as "kind of present, but not inspired by their work or their managers." The remaining 20 percent were actively disengaged. The study also found that disengaged employees were more likely to steal from their companies, negatively influence their coworkers, miss workdays, and drive customers away. Engaged employees usually drove the innovation, growth, and revenue that their companies desperately needed.

It is interesting to me that 70 percent of Americans are classified as overweight or obese, 70 percent of lottery winners are broke within seven years, and 70 percent of American workers are disengaged at work. This tells me that we tend to take the easy way out, to shoot from the hip, if you will. We let life happen to us instead of living a plan to achieve what we want. But I believe we each have what it takes to be successful in every area of life.

The "More" of a Healthy Lifestyle

I've written a couple of times now that a healthy lifestyle is more than just staying fit and eating healthy. Ask someone who is living a healthy lifestyle why they work so hard to be healthy. You will not hear this:

- I love getting up at five a.m. and sweating for an hour before work when it is fourteen degrees outside.

- I cannot stand the taste of chocolate or candy, so it is easy to eat healthy.
- I don't have anything else to do so I work out two hours a day.
- Steamed kale and cauliflower tastes so much better than chocolate cake and ice cream, you have no idea.

What you might hear, though, is this:

- When I get up and work out at five a.m., I feel much more energized for the day. I feel like I have accomplished something before I even get started.
- I know chocolate and candy taste great, but the taste lasts only a moment. I would rather eat healthy and feel great all day.
- I am busy with work, kids, and volunteer activities, but I find time to work out because it relieves my stress and actually gives me the energy to do more.
- Chocolate cake and ice cream are awesome, but they should be consumed only at times of celebration. My body needs the nutrients from fruits and vegetables like kale and cauliflower to work efficiently day in and day out.

These people have a plan. They have a goal and know that working their plan is the tried and true way to achieve it. Even if they have not yet reached their goal, they have tasted success. When you start to truly live a healthy lifestyle you start to see things differently. You gain confidence. You gain self-esteem. You gain your *life*!

Many people get hung up on the "healthy" in "healthy lifestyle" as being difficult to achieve, while it's actually the "lifestyle" piece they're missing. When you say your goal is to lose 50 pounds, what you're really saying is that you want to live the life you envision you will have when you're 50 pounds lighter. That lifestyle is what you're really after, so rather than setting a goal to lose a certain number of pounds, set a goal to do something gloriously fun once you're at a healthy weight – or to simply enjoy life to the fullest!

A Proper Healthy Lifestyle Goal

I am a runner and love coaching runners. But please don't set a goal to lose a certain number of pounds in order to run in your local 5k next season. Why not? I bet you would rather do anything else *right now* than run, so why should your reward for losing weight be something you probably don't even like to do right now? If you participated in any sport in school other than track and/or cross country, running sprints was your coach's go-to punishment for lack of effort. And running will feel like a punishment if achieving your goal is based solely on that "reward."

You can certainly run a 5k when you want to and feel fit enough to do it. It will feel great to support the cause that the race is held for. But when you don't want to get up and go for a training run on a Saturday morning after a stressful work week, you will just end up feeling angry about what's supposed to be rewarding – a psychological impasse.

Here are some better ideas for rewards when you reach your goal:

- Buy a great new wardrobe.
- Go out on the town for a fancy dinner and dancing – in one of those great new outfits!

- Take a weekend trip to the beach and show off your new body.

- Take a weekend trip to a bed and breakfast in the mountains or in wine country.

- Ride the roller coasters at a theme park, which you haven't been able to do because the seats were too small.

- Go to a big sporting event that you have avoided because you could not walk the stairs in the stadium.

- Go skydiving.

Do something you have always wanted to do but didn't because you were too big or too out of shape. What better way to celebrate and motivate yourself than fulfilling a dream? The focus turns from the dreaded 50 pounds you "have" to lose to the fun thing you "get" to do.

I know you might be thinking, "But that reward costs money I don't have." It's hard to envision spending money that's not in the budget on a reward, so try this: Put a dollar amount on your reward. Let's say you want to lose 50 pounds. At $10 per pound lost, that would be $500. Place an envelope, a clothespin, or anything that holds cash somewhere where it will motivate you – like next to the scale in your bathroom or stuck to your bathroom mirror. Every week put $10 per pound in there for the pounds lost that week.

A healthy loss of one or two pounds per week will take six months to a year. Embrace the discipline to not touch that money until you have hit your goal. If you need to, cut a slit in the lid of a glass jar so the money can go in, then glue the lid on the jar. As an added bonus you get to smash the jar open with a hammer when you hit your goal. (Wear safety goggles, please!)

With $500 you can do any of those things in my list of suggestions above. I think you will not only find it motivating, but you will succeed. It's one thing to see the number on the scale going down; it's a whole other thing to see cash piling up. And when both are happening it is the best of both worlds.

CHAPTER 5

IS EXERCISE REALLY IMPORTANT TO A HEALTHY LIFESTYLE?

Do you not know that those who run in a race all run,
but only one receives the prize? Run in such a way
that you may win.
– 1 Corinthians 9:24

As an exercise physiologist, I always enjoy talking with someone who believes they can be completely healthy without exercising. Sorry to burst your bubble, but it's just not possible.

Don't get caught in the trap of thinking that your BMI or the number on your scale defines your health. Those numbers are *indicators* of your health, but if you rely on one specific number to tell you if you're healthy or not, you're missing the point. Numbers are for *tracking your progress* as you work towards a healthy lifestyle. You should keep track of some basic indicators either on your own or with the help of your doctor.

Your Primary Doctor Is Your Friend

I know that most insurance companies do not afford you a lot of time with your doctor when you go for a visit, but they do allow for an annual checkup or physical. Take advantage of that.

Since I am living a healthy lifestyle, my annual checkup is not a time for my doctor to tell me all the changes I need to make to be healthy (you know, that conversation that keeps most people from going to the doctor because they don't want to hear how badly their health has deteriorated). It's a time to talk about best practices to continue living healthy. I know a lot of this information because my job is to coach people to better health, but my doctor evaluates me as one of my coaches. It is not uncommon for him to see something I have overlooked, as I can get on autopilot in some areas and stop progressing.

Always check with your primary doctor before starting an exercise program. No matter what you think you know is going on in your body, your doctor can tell you for sure and make sure that you take any necessary precautions when exercising.

The Dangers of Exercise

It might seem counterintuitive to mention the dangers of exercise when I am a huge proponent of exercise as a part of a healthy lifestyle, but exercise can be very dangerous. It carries with it the potential for injury to a muscle or joint. And unseen dangers can develop inside your body – specifically in your heart and blood vessels.

Going from zero to 60 with an exercise program throws up red flags for any good trainer or coach. I have been there, done that. I spent the summer before my sophomore year in high school not working out as I was supposed to. I went back for the fall semester, acted as if I had done all the work, and within days developed severe dehydration. I was peeing blood in the locker room after my workout. Talk about scared. From that day forward I followed my coach's advice: "Never walk by a water fountain without taking a drink." Today I still live by that advice, but in the form of carrying a 32-ounce refillable water bottle with me everywhere I go.

Follow a proper exercise routine to avoid injury. Get medical clearance from your doctor first, and if you don't know where to start, find a knowledgeable coach or trainer to help you. Interview them to make sure they are a good fit for your personality and what you want to accomplish. You can find information about my coaching programs on my website, www.allinhealthandwellness.com, or you can email me at jerry@allinhealthandwellness.com.

The True Power of Exercise

There is a power to exercise – not just the raw physical power you outwardly see; the power I'm referring to is in your mind. The biggest byproduct of exercising is the power to positively change your mind. That's saying something, since the physical benefits to your body are so well documented. Yes, exercise changes your body in a healthy way, but WOW, how it can change your mind! …unless you ignore it. Your mind is very powerful. It can decide to ignore even the most basic natural benefit you try to provide it. But when you allow exercise to have its true effect, you reap rewards. It is invigorating, therapeutic, stress-relieving, character-building, and confidence-building. It is a basic bodily function that every human being who is not physically challenged can perform. And even if you have physical limitations you still need to move regularly in some way to maintain your health and flexibility.

Unfortunately the word *exercise* gets a bad rap, just like the word *diet*. For some reason, when someone like myself says, "Exercise is important and should be done daily," some people hear, "You have to run a marathon" or "Go to the gym and work until you look like Arnold Schwarzenegger." Of course those thoughts are scary and intimidating. But what I'm really saying is that you should regularly get your heart rate up to what is called the target-heart-rate range (THRR).

Here's some simple math to explain this: 220 beats per minute (bpm) has been determined to be the fastest a human heart should ever beat naturally. (There are drugs that can make it beat faster, but no need to go there.)

Subtract your age from 220 bpm. This is your personal maximum heart rate (MHR) – the fastest your heart should ever beat. (No need to hit this rate unless you are in extremely great physical condition.)

Your personal THRR is 70 to 85 percent of your MHR. For example, for a 40-year-old:

MHR = 180 bpm
THRR = 126-153 bpm

This formula is not gender specific. Men and women get the same effect from the same formula. Your heart is a muscle. It has no idea whether you're a man or a woman. If it did, there would be a heart-transplant waiting list for men and one for women, which is not the case.

Here's the kicker: To truly burn fat you need to be in your THRR for 30 continuous minutes. And I'm sorry to tell you this but the fact that you can't afford a fancy watch with heart rate monitoring capability is not an excuse. God gave you this really cool feature that tells you when you have reached your THRR. It's called sweat!

Oh no, that's another word that scares people. I've heard all of these:

"I would exercise but I don't want to be all sweaty."

"I don't like to sweat."

"When I sweat I feel all sticky and gross."

A little tough love here: get past it. I want you around for as long as possible. That means you have to live healthy by exercising, which means sweating.

You might ask, "But I can walk an hour a day without sweating. That's good exercise, right?" It's great to get out and breathe the fresh air and stretch and improve your flexibility, but if you're not sweating – if you're not sweating for at least 30 minutes – it's not going to get you to optimal health.

You might even say, "But I am losing weight as a result of walking." Yes, you can lose weight by walking an hour a day even without getting into your THRR. Remember, though, that the number on the scale is not the only indicator of good health. (Have you ever heard of a skinny non-smoker having a heart attack? I have.) What is happening is that by sheer volume of movement you are losing weight. But if you're not sweating, you're not flushing the toxins from your blood vessels and organs, therefore chronic diseases are still a major concern.

Why the THRR Is So Important

Think of a garden hose when water is flowing out of it freely and easily. Think of this as your heart when you are at rest. Now imagine putting your thumb on the end of the hose and cutting off the flow as much as possible. The water comes out with a lot more force because pressure has built up in the hose. When you point that fast stream of water at the dirt, it starts to break through the dirt like a hot knife through butter. When you exercise you increase your heart rate – the speed at which blood flows through your blood vessels increases. The additional pressure breaks down deposits in your blood vessels. And your cells burn fuel to keep up with the energy need.

Another benefit is that the waste byproduct of this rapid fuel burn is taken up by the blood cells and delivered to your liver and kidneys to be filtered out of the body, removing those toxins from your body.

There is another way to get your blood to flow like the pressurized water hose; it's called hypertension, or high blood pressure (HBP). We established that your heart is a muscle. HBP makes your heart feel like your legs after a Thanksgiving Day pickup football game with the family – it's fun in the moment but you might not be able to get out of bed for a couple of days because your muscles are so sore.

Your heart and blood vessels cannot handle HBP for long. Your heart will actually develop serious problems – it cannot get out of bed. Which leads to other problems. Think about how ineffective you are when you are so sore you can hardly move. Your family suffers, your job suffers, and you suffer, both physically and emotionally. But if you had been exercising regularly, you would not be sore!

How Does Diet Relate to Exercise?

You might think that if you exercise in your THRR for 30 minutes a day, three to five days a week, you can eat whatever you want to. That depends on your current health. If you are at your target weight and exercising properly, you can splurge more often. It is difficult, though, to exercise efficiently on poor nutrition. As you exercise more your brain starts to naturally crave less-toxic foods, even to the point of being turned off by unhealthy foods. Will you lose the craving for chocolate forever? No. But it will lessen.

I recently had a conversation with a male in his fifties about dietary changes he and his wife made due to her receiving a diagnosis of breast cancer. They decided to cut meat out of their diet almost completely and go heavy on the vegetables and fruits. They began juicing to supplement their nutritional needs. (I recommend this and do this myself.) After three weeks of being on this healthy plan he decided to eat a brand of popsicle that he had loved prior to changing his food regimen. He said he almost instantly felt the difference in the nutritional value compared to the healthy foods he had been eating. He didn't even finish the popsicle, and hasn't touched another one since.

That's what making a simple change can do in your body. When you can feel it like that, you realize just how hard the struggle to maintain your weight is when you do not eat properly, even if you exercise.

There's No Time

We all have 168 hours a week. How many do you need to spend on exercise to be healthy? It depends on your current health and your goals. Once you are at a healthy weight and lifestyle, maintenance can be accomplished with as little as one-and-a-half hours a week.

"Wait. What? One-and-a-half hours a week and I can maintain good health? Why don't I hear that in the news or recommended by the government?" Remember that the majority of Americans are overweight or obese. If you exercise only enough to maintain your current fitness, you are *maintaining* an unhealthy lifestyle. And your internal health is deteriorating every day you don't exercise. It compounds as each day goes by.

You can change that by using just 1.8 percent of your week to exercise. That's three hours to push past the maintenance level. That breaks down to 30 minutes a day, six days a week. Remember, though, that is 30 minutes in your THRR (sweating). Why not shoot for 45 minutes four days a week to provide enough time for a proper warm-up and cool down afterward, while getting 30 minutes of good workout in your THRR.

Why do you hear about recommendations for one hour of exercise a day every day? Because many people never get to their THRR during exercise. The goal of recommending an hour a day is to instill a habit of exercising. By committing to an hour a day you are likely to increase the intensity of your workouts after several days and start to get into your THRR for at least a half hour.

Seven hours a week is a lot for today's busy people, especially when they go from no exercise to seven hours a week. But I don't think you have to exercise seven hours a week to become healthy. That level of exercise at THRR is for people competing in sporting events. It's not for everyone. But exercise is.

I hope it's obvious that no one should go from years of no exercise to a 45-minute THRR workout on day one. A good coach/trainer will keep your first day very simple – stretching and slow exercises with low weight resistance. You might not even get into your THRR on day one, which is okay. Slow and steady wins the race. Learn how to do the exercises with the proper form first. Stretch and get your body used to moving again. Then slowly add resistance and speed to your workout.

It takes time. Remind yourself that you did not create your unhealthy body in one day, so you cannot reverse it in one day. But you can become healthy quicker than you might think with the proper exercise routine and diet.

You Don't Have to Become a Bodybuilder or a Marathoner

Everyone who competes in the games goes into strict training. They do it to get a crown that will not last, but we do it to get a crown that will last forever.

– 1 Corinthians 9:25

We are all supposed to be training our bodies to be in good health. Any athlete preparing for their season does pre-season workouts in which they start with the basics. It's the same for an exercise program when you have been sedentary for years – first things first: make sure you check with your doctor before beginning. You may have a hidden health issue that needs to be addressed before exercise causes that issue to become more serious.

Years ago, before I started my business, my father-in-law decided to get healthy and signed up for a gym membership. He did a few workouts with a personal trainer, and then the trainer heard that he had enjoyed lifting weights in high school when he was a lineman in football. The trainer promptly had him start lifting weights. Within a few days he had pulled a muscle in his arm, was sore all over, and was pretty ticked at the trainer. Needless to say, he cancelled his membership.

I suggest not touching a single weight for weeks, if not months. Unless you want to be a bodybuilder, you do not need to lift weights. You might already have difficulty lifting your own weight, so why add to it? Learn how to lift your own weight, start converting your fat weight to muscle weight, and clean yourself out on the inside.

The first step is building up your core muscles. These are not just the "six pack" abdominal muscles but include muscles in your hips, back, and shoulders. It's like building a house: if you don't spend time on a proper foundation, the house will crumble sooner rather than later. Spend time building your core muscles so that when you later begin building other muscles, your body won't crumble.

One of the easiest ways to tell if you are building your core muscles is if your posture improves. Are you holding yourself up straight in a chair without pain? Are you standing up tall? Those are your core muscles at work. Some basic core exercises are push-ups, leg lifts, dips, various types of crunches, planks, and wall sits. Starting out, you might do the same three to five exercises for four or five days a week, later graduating to a weekly routine with different exercises each day.

Cardiovascular (cardio) exercises should also be included when starting an exercise program. These get your heart rate up and keep it up through continual motion. Examples include vigorous walking, jogging, swimming, cycling, and rollerblading (does anyone do that anymore?). Cardio is the best type of exercise for getting your heart rate into your THRR and keeping it there for 30 minutes at a time to burn fat. But if you don't also work on your core muscles you could injure yourself fairly quickly. Don't try to run for 30 minutes on the first day. Start by walking for maybe five minutes to see how that feels. Increase your walking time by a minute each day. When you feel ready to jog, start back at five minutes again. Don't assume that if you can walk for 30 minutes you can jog for 30 minutes.

Still Not Convinced You Need to Exercise for Your Health?

Maybe I bored you with all the science and math behind what exercise does inside your body. Maybe you think there is still time in the future to take care of that but right now you are too busy. If you're still not sold on it, visit the nearest cardiac rehabilitation clinic. Jenny has worked in cardiac rehab for 20 years and I visit her there often, so I know the scene. In fact, I have a little saying for potential clients when they're not convinced: You can work with me to prevent a cardiac event or work with my wife after a cardiac event.

One way or another (if you live in Waco, Texas), you will be taught how to be healthy by a Snider.

What you will see at a cardiac rehab clinic are some patients who are post heart surgery, some who are pre-surgery, and others who are recovering from a heart attack or stroke. You will see nurses and exercise physiologists instructing patients to exercise properly. You will see grown men struggling to lift two pounds in repetition. You will see women sweating (don't be alarmed!). You will see patients wearing heart monitors and being watched like a hawk. You will see fear in the eyes of new patients; having just been through a life altering event they are fearful will happen again.

You will also see patients who are at the end of their insurance-approved 36 sessions over 12 weeks. They exhibit the joy of having their lives back – the joy of knowing they have a second chance; the "big one" did not kill them. They also show a little fear. Can they continue to live their new healthy lifestyle without the help of the rehab clinic? Twelve weeks of training stacked up against years of bad health habits?

What you will hear if you ask a few questions could be even more profound. Ask about the cost of what they have been through. The average bypass surgery costs well over $100,000 just while you are in the hospital. That does not include rehabilitation and medications; the total costs of a cardiac event can easily reach $200,000 or more. Check your yearly out-of-pocket maximum on your insurance and get ready to pay that amount. Motivated to exercise yet?

Ask a physiologist, "What is one of the most common things patients are concerned about when they start rehab?"

If there's a heart issue in your future, you want to know what the biggest concern is, right? It might surprise you, but one of the top three is when or even if they can have sex again.

We all share the same basic enjoyments. Our hearts beat a little faster during sex, so after going through a life-or-death situation such as a major heart issue you would understandably be concerned about being left behind sexually. Intimacy typically relieves stress in a relationship. The inability to express intimacy through making love can be emotionally devastating for some. It's not just your heart that loses strength, but being in the hospital causes deterioration of your muscles to some degree because you're normally not that inactive. A regular exercise routine is not only a key ingredient in prevention of heart disease, it also ensures you have the strength to bounce back from a hospital stay no matter what the reason for being hospitalized. It's never too late to start an exercise routine. Just check with your doctor before starting to make sure you don't have any hidden medical issues that need to be addressed.

Ready to Start?

It's not complicated, but let's review: Get checked out by your doctor. Find a coach or trainer to help you get started.

Yes, that means paying someone, at least for a while, to get fit safely. It's worth it. After a few months you will find yourself saving money. Contrary to popular belief, it's less expensive to live a healthy lifestyle than not to. In the long run fewer visits to the doctor means your insurance and medical costs will go down. You will learn to eat proper portions, so even though healthy food is more expensive, you won't consume as much and your food costs will go down.

Byproducts of a healthy lifestyle that most people overlook are the confidence it breeds in you and the mental energy you gain, which often means you are more productive at work. That can mean a promotion, an increase in income, or perhaps a whole new exciting career.

Start today. Download my Free Stretching Plan from my website, www.allinhealthandwellness.com, and put your body in motion towards a healthy lifestyle.

CHAPTER 6
MEDICINE AND FOOD

A cheerful heart is good medicine,
but a crushed spirit dries up the bones.

– Proverbs 17:22

The prevalence of medications for everything from a sniffle to erectile dysfunction is an indication that we take our health for granted. Health is an afterthought because we know we can pop a pill to address most any medical problem. It should not be that way. Medicine can and does work, but a healthy lifestyle can prevent many illnesses and resolve many medical conditions. (In this chapter I'm referring only to prescribed medications, not vaccinations.)

Just Take Your Medicine

"Take your medicine; it's good for you." If you are a parent you have probably said this on more than one occasion, especially when your pharmacist forgets to include the bubblegum flavor. But do you really need the quick fix of medication for every little illness and ailment?

Do you truly understand all the potential side effects of every medication you take? That's like asking if you read all the fine print before signing a contract – most people don't. And most people don't understand the potential side effects of the medications they take.

Years ago I was prescribed a nasal spray for allergies. I filled the prescription and took my first dose. I'm so glad Jenny was home when I did, because I almost immediately felt clammy, started sweating, my heart started racing, and I nearly passed out. We grabbed the box and read through the side effects to discover that I was allergic to the medication. Out went the $5/month nasal spray and in came the $65/month version. My wallet was allergic to that one! But at the time I thought I needed it because my allergy symptoms sometimes got very bad.

A few years later I was describing the situation to a new friend. He told me he took a spoonful of local honey every day to prevent his allergies. I thought, "Sixty-five dollars versus a nine-dollar jar of local honey?" I tried the honey. It did not work immediately because it had to build up in my system, but a few weeks later I said goodbye to my nasal spray for good. If you want to try honey for your seasonal allergies, be sure to use local honey. You are allergic to local plants and their pollen. Local honey is produced by local bees using that same pollen that you are allergic to. The honey builds your immunity to the pollen, which is why it takes a few days to take effect.

Avoid medications and supplements that claim to provide weight loss, especially ones that are not FDA approved. There are several diet pills that are approved in other countries but are not deemed safe by our government. That alone should be a red flag. If an expert tells you they are skeptical of one you are considering, you should automatically wonder why. Some of them may actually do what they promise initially, but the long-term side effects are the bigger issue. As one doctor I spoke with about my program said, "Why do something so risky as diet pills or surgery when the tried and true method of exercise and healthy eating works every time?"

Is It Cheaper to Medicate?

You know the look most people get when someone tells them that Brussels sprouts taste great – that "What 'choo talkin' bout, Willis" look from Arnold on *Diff'rent Strokes*. That is the way I look when someone tells me it's cheaper and easier to take medicine than to live healthy from the get-go. Quicker, maybe – because it is going to take some time to reverse all the poor health decisions you made during your life that got you where you are. But it is definitely not less expensive. Even if you have reached your deductible on your insurance plan for the year and you now get free generic medications, *they are not free.* You had to pay insurance premiums to get to where there's no out-of-pocket expense. Just because you can go to the pharmacy, pick them up, and not pay anything does not mean they're free. When you're not healthy you take more medications. So even if you save money on groceries by not buying healthy foods, the expense of medications alone (not to mention healthcare costs) can be more than what you save on groceries.

But It's So Easy to Just Pop a Pill

Sure it's easy to pop a few pills every few hours when you're sick, hoping they will alleviate your discomfort. But do you really know what you're doing to your body? Maybe you've noticed the reams of fine print that come with prescription medications these days describing all the scary side effects. The next time you see a commercial for prescription medication, notice that you can't even read the side effects because of the speed at which they have to flash them on the screen to fit them into the commercial.

"Easy" and "good for you" are two completely different things. Remember, the fast food drive-thru is easy, but rarely if ever good for you. Just as we don't take the time to know what is in the food at fast food places, we don't take the time to read about the side effects of our medications.

It is the winter of 2017-2018 as I'm writing this, and the flu this year is particularly bad. The flu shot has been estimated to be 10 percent effective. One of the most common medicinal remedies for the flu is oseltamivir phosphate, sold under the brand name Tamiflu®, if given within the first two days of the flu diagnosis. Here is a *partial* list of *common* side effects of Tamiflu as reported at https://www.rxlist.com:

- Nausea
- Vomiting
- Diarrhea
- Dizziness
- Headache
- Nosebleed
- Eye redness or discomfort

- Sleep problems (insomnia)
- Cough or other respiratory problems

Now let's look at the symptoms of the flu as reported by the CDC:

- Fever, or feeling feverish/chills
- Cough
- Sore throat
- Runny or stuffy nose
- Muscle or body aches
- Headaches
- Fatigue (tiredness)
- Some people may have vomiting and diarrhea, though this is more common in children than in adults.

If you have the flu and are experiencing headaches, you can take Tamiflu and still have headaches. The flu headaches may be gone but you have replaced them with Tamiflu headaches. And if you're not experiencing headaches, take Tamiflu and you might add them to your list of symptoms!

Tamiflu might get you back to normal a couple of days sooner, but it's not worth the risk of additional symptoms. Medications are rarely completely natural products, and some have no natural substances in them at all. They put extra strain on your liver and kidneys in filtering the medication out of your system. I don't mean to pick on Tamiflu, because many medications come with the same drawbacks; it's just a bad flu season so it was the first one that came to mind.

Your Immune System Should Be Your Best Friend

Building up your immune system is a far better choice than continually taking medications. A healthy diet and exercise does just that. It takes a few weeks, and your immune system can become even weaker before getting stronger, so stay clear of high-traffic areas for a while and be vigilant about washing your hands during this time.

That's why spring is the best season to embark on a healthy lifestyle. New Year's resolutions are popular, and the most popular might be getting healthy, but you don't want to weaken your immune system during the dead of winter when viruses are more prevalent. If you get sick you'll stop exercising. You'll stop eating healthy because nothing stays in you. Your work towards your resolution will go out the window and you'll give up.

If you start in the spring when things are in bloom, when you can exercise outside away from other people, when it's neither too cold nor too hot, when illnesses are not as prevalent, I guarantee you will have better success. You won't have that bikini body or six pack by spring break, but if you haven't exercised for months or years you wouldn't have gotten it by March anyway, so set it as your goal for next year's spring break.

The cool thing is what happens after you make it past that initial drop in your immunity. Your immune system bounces back with a vengeance. You become almost illness-proof, *almost* being the key word. Even if you're in prime health you might still have a hard time fighting off the flu if someone who's infected sneezes in your face, but you will likely not be down and out for as long as someone who is not healthy.

If it's summer now, don't wait until next spring to get healthy! I just want you to be aware that the exertion of starting to exercise and the change in diet can make your system weaker for a short time. If there's a virus going around and you are regularly in contact with people, wait a few weeks or start much more slowly to be sure you stay healthy.

CHAPTER 7

NUTRITIONAL SUPPLEMENTS: VITAMINS, MINERALS, AND SUPERFOODS

*And he humbled you and let you hunger and fed you with
manna, which you did not know, nor did your fathers
know, that he might make you know that man does not live
by bread alone, but man lives by every word that comes
from the mouth of the Lord.*

– Deuteronomy 8:3

All the nutrients we need can come from food, right? Not necessarily. We can need nutritional supplements to get some of the micronutrients that are not available in our "modern" food system.

For many people nutritional supplements are the most confusing part of learning about nutrition. There are hundreds of companies selling supplements. Some of the products are great for you and some are not. But what is even more confusing is that the same product can be great for you but not helpful at all for your spouse or sibling.

I recently met with a 24-year-old guy who has been lifting weights for several years. Although he admitted to not doing enough cardio and not always making the healthy food choice, he is physically fit. When I asked him if he was taking any nutritional supplements, he replied that he was not. He stated he had not done enough research on supplements. He agreed it made sense to take supplements given our current food supply, but he wasn't ready to start putting something in his body that he did not understand. That is a very smart stance to take.

What Is a Nutritional Supplement?

We've probably all been exposed to some type of nutritional supplement whether it be a juice, a shake, a pill, or some other form of product. There are commercials, infomercials, network marketing companies, and retail stores dedicated to selling these products. For most people the first two questions are "What do I start with?" and "Why does it all cost so much?"

Not only am I going to try to answer those questions but I hope to give you enough basic knowledge to determine if you should be taking supplements. First we have to define what a supplement is.

Thefreedictionary.com provides this definition: "Nutritional supplements include vitamins, minerals, herbs, meal supplements, sports nutrition products, natural food supplements, and other related products used to boost the nutritional content of the diet." Basically any such product that is not part of a food group (meats, grains, fruits, etc.) that provides a positive boost to nutrition is a supplement. And I believe that every person needs to supplement their meal plan with one or two products. Sorry, candy does not count.

How Do I Know If I Need to Add a Supplement to My Diet?

One way to find out if you need a supplement is to have a fully comprehensive blood test done. Granted there is a cost involved, but it's the best way to get a complete picture of what is going on inside your body. The caveat is that the results are compared to averages of what doctors and scientists believe are the proper amounts of nutrients to have in your body. Even if the test shows that your level of a particular nutrient is within the average range, it might not be the best level for you as an individual.

A non-invasive way to find out what supplemental nutrients you might need is to complete a health survey with a nutritionist or health coach. A professional can diagnose deficiencies in your diet simply by studying what you eat and how your body reacts. There can be some trial and error in adjusting various nutrients to see what works best. This trial and error to solve one issue can also solve others through improving your nutrient intake.

You can also simply tune in to your body and listen to it. If you crave a food, you are likely craving the nutrients that food provides. For example, if you have a craving for broccoli you could be low in magnesium, iron, or a number of other nutrients that broccoli provides. This isn't the easiest way to determine which supplements to add to your meal plan on a long-term basis, and of course you have to discount cravings for sweets and unhealthy fats.

Where Do I Start?

First let's assume that you have not had a blood test or completed a health survey. You simply want to make sure you are getting proper nutrition. The best thing to do is start with products that contain multiple nutrients. These provide the best bang for your buck.

If you have had a blood test, your physician should be able to tell you exactly what nutrients to add to your diet. Then you have to decide whether to buy only that nutrient or a multi-nutrient product. Cost can be a deciding factor, as most single-nutrient products are less expensive than the multiple versions. But you might not need the high dose that the single packaging provides. For example, a 500mg vitamin C tablet is 833 percent of the recommended daily dose. But you can find vitamin C at 50 or 100 percent of the recommended dose in a multivitamin or another supplement.

A good health survey assesses your total health and activity level, while a blood test is a single-point-in-time measurement. While blood tests are good for pinpointing issues, assessing your total lifestyle provides a more comprehensive result. A knowledgeable health professional can help you adjust your meal plan to improve your nutrient intake through food while supplementing with certain nutrients to address any other issues.

What Are Superfoods?

Superfoods are not a new concept, but the label "superfood" is new. These are foods that are dense in nutritional value. They naturally contain a lot of vitamins, minerals, and antioxidants that your body needs. An *antioxidant* is a substance that inhibits oxidation, such as those used to counteract the deterioration of stored food products. They prevent non-nutritional food ingredients from damaging your cells.

Most superfoods are plant-based. (Sorry, guys, but you really do need to eat your vegetables.) You have a choice to make: Spend hundreds of dollars a month on nutritional supplements to acquire the vitamins and minerals you need, or eat the proper fruits and vegetables along with spending just a few dollars a month on supplements.

Examples of superfoods include foods you are already familiar with and some you have probably never heard of: quinoa, blueberries, kale, chia seeds, flax seeds, matcha green tea, strawberries, broccoli, almonds, beets, ginger, ashwagandha, and cacao are just a few. They provide the necessary vitamins, minerals, antioxidants, and amino acids that your body needs. They're all grown from the earth, but you won't be able to find all of them in your local grocery store. And be careful about buying them in concentrated pill form because they can lose potency depending on how they are processed and prepared.

How Do I Know If It's Working?

Are you getting any benefits or are you just spending money? If you are truly deficient in what you're supplementing, you should notice a change in your energy level, focus, and performance. This change might take a week or two to show up depending on the nutrient and how deficient you are when you start taking it. If you do not see or feel a change, consult the person who recommended the supplement for further suggestions.

It is possible to take too much of a given nutrient, but it rarely causes negative side effects. Most excess nutrients are filtered out of your body by your kidneys. If you notice that your urine is bright yellow or green, you're probably taking more than you need. Green urine is an indicator of a diet high in sugar. You should definitely question the sugar content of the supplement if you experience green urine. You should not be paying for sugar in your supplements, and if you're excreting excess nutrients, that's also costing you money unnecessarily spent.

The key to knowing if it's working is to first know what the supplement is supposed to do. Is it supposed to give you energy, help you sleep better, or help you focus? If you don't know what it's supposed to do, you won't be able to tell if it's working.

Proceed with Caution

Each person is a little different, so I can't advise you about any particular supplement without specifics about your situation. There are a lot of good supplements on the market but there are also some that are low-quality or essentially worthless. As mentioned, beware of supplements with high sugar content. And avoid anything containing high fructose corn syrup.

I typically recommend multi-nutrient supplements that have high vitamin content and amino acids. These are two nutrient groups that are commonly lost during the processing of foods. Be careful about liquid supplements with long shelf lives, as many lose potency after only a week on the shelf.

Be wary of someone trying to sell you a supplement that you cannot try first. We don't expect to be able to taste-test items in a big-box grocery store, but small nutrition stores usually let you try before you buy. People who promote nutritional supplements via network marketing companies always let you try a sample before committing to a large bottle. It takes at least 48 hours to feel an effect from a nutritional supplement, and even a couple of weeks for certain kinds, so don't buy a month's supply before you've determined that it works. Ask the salesperson how long it should take to notice the effect.

A friend once tried to sell me his vitamin water. He said it would instantly balance my body's pH and I would feel stronger. Before I tried it he had me do a balance test while trying to knock me over. He succeeded in making me tilt my body. I took one drink of the vitamin water and we tried again. This time I was able to hold myself up. What had actually happened was that my mind now knew what to expect and I subconsciously braced myself better, therefore keeping my balance. So I did not buy his expensive water. He is still a friend, though. Never let business come between friends.

I hope this helps you navigate the world of supplements. Remember to ask questions before you try or buy anything. Supplements can be a great investment but they can also be a waste of money if you don't educate yourself about them. For a look at the supplements I use, visit my website, www.allinhealthandwellness.com.

CHAPTER 8

THE QUESTION OF ALCOHOL

Wine is a mocker and beer a brawler;
whoever is led astray by them is not wise.

–Proverbs 20:1

I believe that alcohol can be a part of living a healthy lifestyle, though it does present challenges (not to mention the dangers of alcoholism and driving under the influence). You can accomplish weight loss and still enjoy a tasty adult beverage on occasion. Of course the most effective way to deal with alcohol during a weight-loss program is to completely abstain from it. Short of abstaining, you should always consume alcohol in moderation. Drinking to get drunk is not at all a part of a healthy lifestyle.

Wine, beer, and liquor each present a different issue if you are attempting to lose weight.

Wine

There is research that showed that wine provided both positives and negatives for health. It has long been thought that red wine helps prevent coronary artery disease, which causes heart attacks. It makes sense because wine comes from grapes and grapes are a healthy food product.

A glass of wine a few nights a week also helps with stress relief. It's just enough to take the edge off, per se. Reducing stress helps reduce the effects of heart disease in your body and improves your outlook on life, so it can certainly contribute to a healthy lifestyle.

But wine, especially sweet wine, is high in sugar. Many people experience bloating the day after drinking wine, especially as they age. This is a negative because fluid retention puts extra stress on your heart.

Red wines are thought to have the biggest health benefit. An antioxidant called resveratrol is found in red wine and has been shown to help lower cholesterol and reduce blood clots. Resveratrol comes from the skin of the grape, which is used during fermentation of red wines. Research is still being done on these effects.

Moderation is always key with any kind of alcohol. One 5-ounce glass of red wine a day is plenty if you are seeking health benefits from it. (https://www.mayoclinic.org/diseases-conditions/heart-disease/in-depth/red-wine/art-20048281?pg=1)

Beer

Most beers don't have as much alcohol content as wine or liquor, but that is not necessarily a good thing. It means you can drink more before feeling the intoxicating effect. There is a lot of research that showed both positive and negative effects of beer on health.

It has been well documented that consuming several beers on a daily basis can negatively affect your liver. (https://www.livestrong.com/article/392731-liver-health-and-beer) You can also experience kidney issues. But there is a bigger issue: Beer and junk food go together in our society. You do not typically see beer sold at health food restaurants. Obviously not every restaurant that serves beer is automatically an unhealthy place to eat, but restaurateurs know that if they serve you beer you will likely eat more. And when you become inebriated your portion control goes out the window.

Beer is also considered empty calories. Why do you think there are all those commercials emphasizing the calorie count of beer? But brewers are in the business of making the best-tasting beer they can, not the lowest-calorie beer.

What is really cool about living a healthy lifestyle is that when I want to partake in a beer, I don't have to choose a low-calorie one. I can drink the one that tastes best to me, or try a new one, but I never worry about the calorie count. I know my exercise routine will work those empty calories off before they get a chance to do any real damage.

Liquor

Most liquors are lower in calories than wine and beer, so that's the healthy choice, right? Not really. Most have a higher alcohol content than wine or beer, so while one shot of vodka is lower in calories than a glass of wine, it relaxes you faster, making it harder to stay on your healthy plan.

The real issue liquor presents to a healthy lifestyle is the mixed drink. Most mixers double or triple the calorie count of the liquor alone. Margaritas are a popular drink in my state of Texas. One frozen margarita with a salted rim can contain nearly a third of the calories you need to consume on a given day, coming in at 500 to 600 calories. That is a lot of empty calories, and if you are having that margarita with a meal you will likely consume all your calories for the day in one sitting, because a typical enchilada dinner comes in at over 1,100 calories. The drink and dinner plate total 1,700 calories even without chips and salsa, an appetizer, a dessert, and a refill of that margarita. (https://www.eatthismuch.com/food/view/enchilada-dinner) Your body is not meant to consume and process that many calories all at one time. God created us to process calories throughout the day, not in one hour. How will you fuel yourself for the next 23-plus hours in a healthy way after such a meal?

Short-Term Sacrifice for Long-Term Gain

Alcohol relaxes your mind, which is one of the reasons so many people have a drink after a tough day at work. Happy hour is a time to come together with friends and relax. But it also relaxes your resistance to impulsive behavior. While you do not have to abstain from alcohol to lose weight, it does make sticking to your healthy plan easier. Instead of reaching for that beer to reduce stress, go for a walk. Do 15 minutes of conditioning exercises. Go to a yoga class. Not only will you reduce your stress through exercise, you will burn calories instead of consuming them. Once you reach a healthy weight and have a truly healthy lifestyle you can add alcohol back into your diet; just do so in moderation. Just as alcohol makes it more difficult to stay on your plan to lose weight, it has the same effect on maintaining your healthy weight.

CHAPTER 9
FASTING

This calls for patient endurance on the part of the people of God who keep his commands and remain faithful to Jesus.

– Revelation 14:12

Fasting is abstaining from all or some kinds of food or drink, especially as a religious observance. It has been practiced since the time of Moses. In biblical days fasting was a part of religious rituals. Today it is still practiced in religious circles to become closer to God. It is also gaining momentum as a way to control weight.

Members of my high school wrestling team fasted in order to make weight for tournaments. I specifically remember John, who spent almost an entire day running laps around the school track in sweats, without any water or food, trying to shed a few pounds so he could compete at his weight class. He accomplished his goal, and I think he even lost a few extra pounds. I don't remember whether he won or lost his match, but I remember he was very lethargic the next day.

All-Day Fasting

When I initially hear that someone is thinking about fasting, my first question is "How *hangry* do you get?" Of course they will get *hungry* – their body needs food; so their tolerance of fasting will depend on their ability to prevent feeling hangry. *Hangry* is used to describe being so hungry that you become angry. While the physical state of being hangry is a true physiological response to hunger, controlling the outward emotion of anger is easier for some than it is for others.

You probably know someone who gets hangry. Jenny gets hangry at times. She knows it. I know it. Her boss and coworkers know it. It's part of her body's reaction to hunger. And there is nothing wrong with it as long as you can control your anger. If you are hangry on a regular basis you need to either eat more often or eat more nutritious meals – your body is talking to you.

Fasting all day will likely cause you to become hangry to some extent. To deal with it, fasters focus on the reason behind their fast, be it religious, political, raising awareness, or personal improvement. Make sure your reason is solid enough to maintain the will power to finish the fast. I also recommend a little self-promotion with friends and coworkers. Fasting is easier when your coworker does not ask you to buy a box of Girl Scout cookies from their daughter. Is there a more tempting item on the planet than Thin Mints? I think not.

Intermittent Fasting

We have all skipped a meal because we were too busy to stop and eat or due to illness. The difference between skipping a meal or two and intermittent fasting is whether or not you do so on purpose.

An intermittent fast can be beneficial if you make sure that the meals you do eat provide enough nutrition-rich calories for the tasks of your day. As with all-day fasting, it takes awareness of your body to make sure you don't trigger starvation mode, and you should keep your emotions in check. If you have a particularly stressful or emotional day when skipping lunch, you can end up bingeing at your evening meal and more than make up for the calories you missed at lunch.

Does Fasting Work for Weight Loss?

Remember the weight-loss formula:

Calories Out – Calories In = Weight Change

So yes, if you severely limit calories you will eventually lose weight. But as discussed in chapter 3, remember to be very careful about consuming fewer calories than your basal metabolic rate dictates you need to keep you alive.

Fasting is not an ideal strategy when trying to establish long-term healthy habits. Unless you deal with the subconscious food cravings that brought you to your unhealthy state, the likelihood of those habits returning after you stop fasting is high. In this regard fasting is no better than a fad diet.

We can all agree that exercising increases the "Calories Out" part of the formula. So exercising combined with fasting should rapidly increase weight loss. But while you might lose weight rapidly over the first few days, exercising while fasting is dangerous because in the absence of proper fuel your body uses its stored fat for fuel, which is lower in nutritional value than a healthy meal. This makes you prone to injury, especially bone injuries such as stress fractures. It can even lead to serious organ malfunction and a hospital stay.

So I don't recommend fasting as a weight-loss strategy. I do, however, support those who fast for religious or personal reasons. Gandhi comes to mind as someone who fasted as a political activist. Fasting can raise awareness of an unethical or inhumane situation. It can also bring a group of people together for a cause or as a means of intentional group prayer. These are all very valid reasons for fasting, but be very cautious about exercising during times of fasting.

While not due to fasting, I have experienced stress fractures on three different occasions in my 30 years of running. Stress fractures are painful, but the worst part is you simply cannot do any exercise that causes stress to the bone until it heals – no running, limited walking, limited everything – and it is very difficult to maintain proper health without exercise. As a result of my most recent stress fracture I gained about 10 pounds over the 12 weeks of extremely limited exercise. That shows that lack of exercise, even while following a very healthy meal plan, can affect one's weight. Because I was at a very healthy weight to begin with, it didn't hurt much to gain that weight and I lost it quickly after I recovered. But imagine my risk for a stress fracture had I been fasting!

CHAPTER 10
DIET VERSUS MEAL PLAN

So whether you eat or drink or whatever you do,
do it all for the glory of God.
— 1 Corinthians 10:31

A healthy lifestyle requires not only eating healthy foods and getting the proper nutrients, but exercising as well. Several clients have asked why they didn't lose weight after years of eating a healthy diet. They were of course missing the exercise piece. Their experiences prove that eating healthy is great but a healthy lifestyle is not based on food alone.

Redefining the Word *Diet*

My initial conversations with prospective clients include the word *diet* and the terms *meal plan* and *food prep*. They don't like those terms, and even say things like "I do not want to do another diet. I just want to be healthy."

You know that being at your ideal weight is good for you, but you have probably been conditioned to think that dieting means you are going to be miserable. As a child you probably watched adults who dreaded having to go on a diet, which became a self-fulfilling prophecy: the experience was dreadful. In the mind-over-matter battle to change your lifestyle, your mind is already winning before you even pick up your weapon.

Try telling the next person you see that you are going to go on a diet to get healthy. Pay close attention to their reaction and the words they use. More than likely they will ask what type of food you have to give up. They might mention a diet they went on that was successful for a short time but did not work long term. They might encourage you, but if you read their face you will probably see doubt and despair. They think dieting is hard and that you will fail like most people.

But you don't have to think that way! Before you begin transitioning to a healthy lifestyle, address your fear of the word *diet*.

Repeat after Me: Meal Plan

What if you simply stopped using the word *diet* altogether. What if you stopped adding *healthy* in front of it to make it sound more appetizing? Use *meal plan* instead. Chances are you don't have any preconceived notions about *meal plan*. Now you are able to take the first shot in the mind-over-matter battle to change your life.

A diet is simply a plan for eating your meals. Most Americans don't plan their meals because with all the other plans we have to keep up with in our daily lives a meal plan is just one more time-consuming task. But you will be more productive, have more energy, and be less stressed if you plan healthy meals, and all those other plans will become easier to maintain. You can achieve more goals in other areas of your life *if* you take care of your health first.

Practical Tips for Successful Meal Planning

You will find sample meal plans in the next chapter, but be thinking about these tips.

Cook Ahead

Preparing food ahead of time so you can stick to your healthy meal plan takes the guesswork out of a busy schedule. Simply cook your meals for the week on your days off. You can make two or three large dishes and portion them into containers for each meal. Label them and put them in the refrigerator or freezer depending on how long they'll stay fresh. It's that simple.

Jenny prepares our meals each night for the next day. She gets her breakfast ready and puts it in the refrigerator because she often leaves before 6:00am. This allows her to get just a few more minutes of sleep each night. She also preps her lunch for the next day. She works in an outpatient cardiac rehabilitation clinic connected to a family practice doctor's office. If you have ever worked at a doctor's clinic you know that they have lunch catered almost every day by a pharmaceutical company, medical device company, or the likes thereof, a tactic to get the doctors to prescribe their medications. The food is often not particularly healthy. Jenny knows that if she does not take a healthy lunch she risks either skipping a meal (really bad, because she gets hangry) or eating the catered meal. Yes, it's a free meal, but free is not always good, and this is a great example of it.

I am fortunate to work from home, which makes dealing with food cravings pretty easy. I don't work a standard schedule; sometimes I meet clients at 5:30am and sometimes I'm up at 10:00pm writing a client's exercise prescription. This allows me the time to do our grocery shopping during the day when I can avoid the crowds. The time savings is great, but the reduced stress of not dealing with the crowds is probably even more important. Stress leads to poor judgment, and shopping when you're hungry or stressed should be avoided at all costs.

I always shop using our meal plan for the coming days. I admit we are a bit routine when it comes to meals. We have found what meals work for us and we stick with them. Others might think our meal plan lacks variety, but if it works, why stray from it? We're healthy inside and out; there is no reason to change, though we do change things up from time to time based on the season and what is available.

Your Desk Is Not a Table

Get up from your desk and go to the office cafeteria, breakroom, or a park to eat. Don't use the conference room unless you never go in there to conduct business. If you conduct business in the room, don't eat in the room. Even though I work at home I leave my desk and go to another part of the house – usually the kitchen – to eat lunch.

First, you need a mental break from work. Get away from your computer even if, like me, you eat quickly. Unless I am meeting with someone at lunch I tend to eat in less than 10 minutes. Even if it's short, you need a break from work.

Second, if you eat at your desk with your work all around you, answering emails or working on a project, you associate the pressures of work with your food, or vice versa. This interferes with the process of enrichment that fueling your body provides. Over time you associate eating with stress, not only at lunch but at other meals as well, which is the opposite of the mindset you want while nourishing your body.

And when you eat at your desk during a busy work day you tend to eat either too quickly or too slowly. When you eat too quickly your stomach and your brain don't have time to communicate about what is happening. You might eat a proper portion, but since your brain has not yet been told you are full, you go to the vending machine and get a snack. Now you are overeating at lunch, not to mention how unhealthy that vending-machine snack most likely is. Get ready for that crash come mid-afternoon.

Be careful not to eat too slowly, though. Your stomach can tell your brain to stop being hungry because "maybe that was just a snack – let's wait for the real meal in a few hours." And if your food gets cold and/or stale, it no longer feels like sustenance and you'll likely throw it out and end up at the vending machine in the mid-afternoon. Time and time again I have seen coworkers eat at their desk only to get interrupted by work, emails, or a phone call. Thirty minutes turns into an hour or more. When they finally get the chance to get back to their lunch, it has been sitting on their desk getting cold and it ends up in the trash.

Try to refrain from eating in your car – at any time, not just during your lunch break. It's messy, and of course driving while eating is dangerous. If you're a salesperson and your car is your office, treat it like your desk and do not eat there.

Eating in your car on a regular basis can also condition you to be hungry when you get into your car, like Pavlov's dog. Now you have trained yourself to need food when you drive. Let me guess – you're going to get those baby carrots and some almonds, because those are easy to eat while driving. ...Oh no, you are going for the chicken nuggets, French fries, chips, and candy, because those are also easy to eat while driving. Remember those restaurant signs on every corner. They are not advertising kale salads, are they? See how quickly you can be trained to eat poorly?

Portion Control

Have you been to both a small hometown restaurant and an uptown classy restaurant lately? If so, you likely noticed a difference, not in just the type of meals offered but in the size of the meals, too. Small local restaurants (especially Mexican restaurants!) give you a large portion of food, practically double what your meal should be. Not to mention the rolls or chips and salsa served as a complimentary appetizer. Whereas at the upscale restaurant you're likely to see more plate than food. They typically provide perfectly sized portions that leave you satisfied even though you paid quite a bit more than you would have at the hometown restaurant.

Portion control is a huge piece of a healthy meal plan, and knowing how and when to stop is easier than you think. It's tied to the type of food you are eating and how quickly you eat. Foods like vegetables and fruits are full of nutrients, low in calories, and take up space in your stomach. While there are suggested portion sizes for vegetables, I contend that you cannot eat too much healthily prepared vegetables – your stomach gets full before you consume too many calories to worry about. If you eat enough French fries to fill your stomach, the calories consumed are wasted because there are simply not enough nutrients in a fried potato.

Here's a simple comparison given that the average adult stomach can hold a volume of about 4.25 cups:

4.25 cups of mixed vegetables have roughly 500 calories.

4.25 cups of French fries from a typical fast food restaurant have roughly 1,000 calories.

Would you rather fill up on the high-nutritional-value vegetables or the high-calorie, non-nutritional French fries?

What if you eat too fast and overeat on vegetables? That doesn't seem like such a bad thing looking at the calorie count, does it? How many of us eat our fast food meal and then take a "daddy tax" from our children's meals – taking some of your kids' food simply because it's owed to you as the dad? I know you are out there because I've done the same thing myself.

Portion control is a life or death decision at every meal. Eating a proper portion size is choosing a healthy life. Eating portions that are more than you need leads to obesity, which is the leading cause of many diseases, including heart disease, which is the leading cause of death in the US and has been for years.

Dealing with Food Allergies

My daughter has been allergic to corn for several years now, and corn is in almost every processed food item. Here are all the ways corn and corn byproducts are used in foods:

- Corn flour, cornmeal, corn gluten, corn flakes
- Cornstarch, also listed on labels as starch or vegetable starch
- Corn oil

- Corn syrup, or high fructose corn syrup
- Dextrins
- Maltodextrins
- Dextrose
- Fructose or crystalline fructose
- Hydrol, treacle
- Ethanol
- Free fatty acids
- Maize
- Zein
- Sorbitol

But even a corn allergy can be overcome by replacing the nutrients that come from that product, either through other foods or nutritional supplements.

Jenny developed an allergy to bananas in the last few years. You've likely heard that bananas are rich in potassium, but there are other foods rich in potassium as well. Jenny simply eats avocados, spinach, and sweet potatoes to meet her potassium needs.

If you believe you have a food allergy, first talk with your doctor. They can perform a test to see what food allergies you have. Question also if the food item could have been exposed to pesticides. There are several studies being conducted to determine if there is a link between pesticides and food allergies. This potential link is driving a push for organic foods. Organic foods typically contain fewer toxins than nonorganic. But you can get the same nutrients from nonorganic foods; you simply have to filter out a few more toxins during the process of digestion.

CHAPTER 11

MEAL PLANS AND NUTRITIONAL GUIDANCE

"I have the right to do anything,"
you say – but not everything is beneficial.
"I have the right to do anything" –
but not everything is constructive.
– 1 Corinthians 10:23

Meal Plans

Be careful about using a meal plan from a book or an online source. If you have not been evaluated by a health coach, doctor, dietician, nutritionist, or physiologist, you can wind up choosing a plan that will not benefit you. As I discussed in previous chapters, dietary needs are different for each of us depending on our gender, age, current weight, and health goals, among other things. Please consult someone knowledgeable about a proper, healthy diet before starting any meal plan.

Having said that, I will provide you with a few examples of what a healthy meal plan looks like. I allow my clients flexibility when following a plan I have provided. I understand that for someone not used to a regimented meal plan it sounds very strict; but in reality it's not.

My tastes and your tastes differ, so I don't provide recipes. I like spicy foods but most of the time we cook with as little seasoning as possible to accommodate the kids. I add a little Jeanpierre's Season-All no-salt-added Cajun seasoning to my food after it's cooked. (That's a little plug for my friend's business. It is really good!) The meal plans I provide are sent on a weekly basis via email. They change from week to week as my clients move from poor eating habits to eating healthy meals. I don't ask clients to give up too many foods at once. While it is good to give up the bad stuff, going step by step allows them to fight cravings one at a time.

I focus on portion control. You will see "normal" food in these meal plans. You will see natural food. You might see more food than you are used to eating, especially if you have a habit of skipping meals. This is a starting point. You will be most successful if you don't try to make a lot of drastic changes at the beginning. If you have spent years creating a craving for a certain food, it will not go away in a day or a week. If everything you eat lacks nutritional value, going cold turkey into a fully healthy meal plan will be very difficult both physically and emotionally. This is where the help of an accountability partner comes in.

The first time I prescribed a meal plan for a client, he started on a Monday and called me on Thursday desperately hungry. I pointed out that this was due to his years of overeating and his addiction to salty foods. He kept with it, and at the end of the first week he had lost five pounds. Yes, he was exercising as well, but he had been exercising for several weeks before going on the meal plan. His weight loss had plateaued, which is why I prescribed the meal plan. I tweaked the plan slightly for the following week. I checked in with him on Thursday of that week and he stated that he was having difficulty eating all the food at each meal. It took about 10 days for his body to reset to eating normal portions of food. He continued to lose weight at a healthy one or two pounds per week while on the meal plan.

So let's take a look at a sample day from one of my meal plans. This is all you are allowed to put in your mouth during the day other than at least a gallon of water throughout the day:

Breakfast:	1 egg, 2 strips bacon, 1 toast w/jelly, glass of 100% OJ or apple juice
10:00am:	apple
Lunch:	grilled chicken salad, no dressing
3:00pm:	banana
Dinner:	salad, 6 oz. meat, 1/2 cup vegetable x 2, 1/2 cup rice
Dessert:	orange (30 minutes after dinner and at least an hour before bed)

This is a meal plan for someone who is just starting out on a healthy lifestyle. I don't go into detail about what type of bacon – turkey bacon, fat free bacon, fully fat bad-for-you bacon; the point is portion control – only two pieces. A few weeks into the plan is when I address the need to switch from bad-for-you bacon to leaner options. I also include fruit juice, which is packed with sugar compared to a piece of fruit. But if you're used to drinking soda all the time, juice can help you transition to a healthy meal plan without craving so much soda.

One of the most common objections I hear is "What about my coffee?" Some of my friends joke with me that I don't let people drink coffee because I have never liked it. But it is more about the stuff you put in your coffee. If you drink it black, have at it. If you put any creamer or sweetener in your coffee you will sabotage your efforts. Think back to the discussion about soft drinks in chapter 2; the sweeteners used in soft drinks are the same sugar substitutes used in products for sweetening coffee. Please avoid these products, in addition to avoiding plain sugar and plain milk.

There is research that showed that a full 16-ounce glass of water first thing in the morning does more to wake you up than coffee. You don't drink while you're asleep, so naturally you're dehydrated when you get up. A big glass of water (you can put a little lemon in it if you like) is what your body is craving. A cup of coffee, which has been shown to have diuretic properties, potentially dehydrates you further. (https://www.livestrong.com/article/485228-green-tea-latte-benefits)

Here is another sample meal plan:

Breakfast:	3/4 cup cereal (don't add sugar) with almond milk (Cheerios, Wheaties, Total), glass of matcha green tea
10:00am:	banana
Lunch:	ham and cheese sandwich on wheat bread, with veggies, OR grilled chicken Caesar salad
3:00pm:	apple or ½ cup raw nuts
Dinner:	6 oz. meat or 8 oz. fish, 1/2 cup vegetable x 2, 1/2 cup rice OR 1/2 cup pasta
Dessert:	orange

This is also for someone just starting out. Portion sizes are based on fueling your body until the next meal. As always, you should exercise in addition to following the plan.

Proper snacks are vitally important because they help regulate your body's glucose level. If your glucose falls too low you get cravings, which are rarely for super healthy foods, so be sure to eat the snacks – don't skip them.

Adding nutritional supplements to this meal plan is simple. If you want to add a juice that's formulated as a dietary supplement, drink it at the time of day that the manufacturer recommends. Depending on what is in the juice and the desired effect, there is a best time of day to drink it. For instance, I drink a juice that contains nutrients for focus and clarity. I drink it around breakfast time each day so I can focus early on the tasks of the day. It should be obvious that you should not drink an energy juice right before you go to bed.

I also drink a protein shake as a meal replacement. I typically do that for lunch during the week and for breakfast on the weekends. Choose your least nutritious meal of the day to replace with a protein shake. If that's breakfast, eat something with a little fiber or physical substance in addition to your shake, since you have not eaten since dinner the previous day, like a piece of fruit, a hard-boiled egg, or some raw nuts.

Nutritional Guidance

Here are my basic nutritional guidelines:

- Drink one gallon of water every day.
- Drink organic superfood juices; almond, soy, or cashew milk; and green teas.

- No more than two cups of coffee a day, without additives.
- Avoid sodas even if you're not trying to lose weight.
- Avoid "energy drinks" (they cause gallstones and kidney stones).
- Avoid fried food.
- Avoid fast food (fresh sandwich-shop sandwiches with lots of veggies are okay).
- Do not use BBQ sauce, ketchup, mayo, salad dressing, or similar sugary condiments.
- Do not add salt to your food ever again.
- Eat three pieces of fresh fruit per day, whether as snacks or with meals.
- Eat 1/2 cup of raw almonds twice a day as a snack.
- Do not use butter or oil to grease your pan. Use coconut-oil spray.
- When you find yourself hungry, drink a glass of water before resorting to a snack.
- Try to consume no more than two processed foods per day (pastas, crackers, items with long shelf-lives).

It's okay if something doesn't work out for you. Don't get down on yourself if you slip up and your salad is served with dressing on it. Just do the best you can. These are goals, not laws, and change is hard. The more you meet the goal the easier it is to make it a lifestyle change, but a slip-up here or there won't derail your long-term plan.

Do not be yoked together with unbelievers. For what do righteousness and wickedness have in common? Or what fellowship can light have with darkness?

– 2 Corinthians 6:14

A very common issue is that one spouse is ready to try a healthy meal plan but the other is stuck on meat and potatoes. Sorry, guys, but there is more out there than meat and potatoes. In the spirit of the verse above, spouses should work together on the same meal plan. If eating healthy is good for one person it's good for the other one as well, especially if one needs to get to a healthy weight. Have your spouse read this book and do your best to convince them to join you on your journey to a healthy lifestyle.

CONCLUSION

If your brother or sister is distressed because of what you eat, you are no longer acting in love. Do not by your eating destroy someone for whom Christ died.

— Romans 14:15

Living a healthy lifestyle has been called:

- A journey
- Something you practice
- A goal to be accomplished

A healthy lifestyle is a journey. It is a destination to be reached. The difficult piece is that once you reach it you have to work to maintain it. With every journey in life there are twists and turns. You've probably heard the adage "The shortest distance between two points is a straight line." But a journey is rarely a straight line. Expect to have difficulty along the way, because you will.

A healthy lifestyle is something you practice. Practice makes perfect, right? Being healthy takes practice, and sometimes lots of it. It takes discipline, which you obtain through practice. Think of your meals at home as practice for eating out at parties. If you are unable to eat and enjoy healthy foods at home you are less likely to stay clear of danger-foods at parties; you will fall in line with everyone else eating multiple cookies and slices of cake. With discipline comes strength. With strength comes perseverance. With perseverance comes accomplishment. With accomplishment comes joy and happiness.

A healthy lifestyle is a goal to be accomplished. Don't put off starting down the path to reach this goal. The faster you accomplish a healthy lifestyle, the more benefit you receive from it. You will see a return on your investment in your health in all areas of your life. The biggest return you receive is self-confidence.

You are in control of how your life plays out – every piece of your life. Once you understand that, it's easier to change the pieces you want to change when you want to change them.

Being healthy starts in your mind, addressing the preconceived notions you have about yourself and how you interact with food and exercise. You get to decide that, not the food. As a society we have settled for quick and easy food for several decades now, but your body subconsciously craves the high-quality nutrients found in good, healthy foods.

Think about other areas of your life. The quick and easy way seldom works out the best. Anything worthwhile takes time, effort, and hard work. Commit to working hard to be healthy. Quick and easy temptations are around you all the time, and a committed, disciplined, healthy lifestyle is the only way to avoid the unhealthy food temptations in our world.

The Formula for Success

Calories Out – Calories In = Weight Change

It seems so simple. But it is so complex. That is what a healthy lifestyle is: complex. It is not too hard to accomplish. It is not impossible. It is complex.

Isaac Newton determined that a body stays in motion until acted upon by an outside force. Your poor eating habits will continue to lead you down an unhealthy path until one of two things occurs: you determine you have had enough and change to a healthy lifestyle; or your body fails in the form of a heart attack, cancer, organ failure, an injury, or another of the many maladies that unhealthy living can surprise you with.

You have to act. Plain and simple. No one else can do it for you. Everyone who loves you will support you. Whomever you enlist as an accountability partner will walk the journey with you.

Exercise is work. You have to work for your body. No one is going to give you a healthy body. It is the most outward result of your decisions. Everyone you meet will instantly know that you are working to be healthy.

The comforting part of the process is that the formula works for everyone, every time. That is not to say that achieving a healthy lifestyle is equally difficult for everyone; we all have our unique personal struggles and temptations. When you overcome your temptations the formula will work for you.

Nobody said achieving your goals would be easy. It is that way for all goals, in all areas of life. You have to do the work.

In fact, avoiding the work makes reaching the goal nearly impossible. Go to work and make your goal happen!

I want to hear from you while you are on your journey. Email me at jerry@allinhealthandwellness.com or message me on my Facebook page, www.facebook.com/allinhealthandwellness, to let me know about your progress. I would love to help you find your motivation.

Focus on your plan. Drink water. Eat healthy. Exercise.

YOU CAN DO THIS! I know you can. Now it's up to *you* to know you can!

Remember, you are never a failure until you quit. Resist discouragement and finish the race God has set before you.

When I was in high school I was coached and mentored by one of the greatest men to walk the planet, Pete Boudreaux. He was my cross country and track coach. He turned 50 when I was a senior, and he is still coaching today, in his seventies. His teams have won an amazing 47 state titles in 50 years of coaching cross country, indoor track, and outdoor track in Louisiana. During cross country season he would constantly remind us of 10 two-letter words to live by. Think of these words when you're in bed and don't want to get up to exercise; think of them when you're out on the town with friends; think of them when you're home alone feeling the pull of ice cream; think of them often and be joyful of your healthy lifestyle: "If it is to be, it is up to me!"

But those who hope in the LORD will renew their strength.
They will soar on wings like eagles; they will run and not
grow weary, they will walk and not be faint.

– Isaiah 40:31

LAGNIAPPE

For physical training is of some value, but godliness has value for all things, holding promise for both the present life and the life to come.

– 1 Timothy 4:8

If you have never lived in South Louisiana, you are probably not familiar with the word *lagniappe*. It means bonus or extra credit. In my school we never had the opportunity to earn "extra credit"; we earned lagniappe. It's pronounced "lan-yap."

In the spirit of lagniappe, I want to share a gift I received in my best friend Christen's house just after graduating from high school. I had grown up in a Catholic home. I attended St. Aloysius, a private Catholic school, from kindergarten through eighth grade. I went on to Catholic High School in Baton Rouge, an all boys' private school.

Getting into Catholic High was the first time I can point to when God truly moved in a miraculous way in my life. I wanted to go there because it was *the* school for sports, and my life at the time revolved around sports. During track practice one day when I was in eighth grade, my track coach, Coach Booth, asked me where I was going to go to high school. I told him my dad said I couldn't go to Catholic High because of the cost, so it was either the magnet school or the local public school. My older sister attended the magnet school, but it didn't have much of a sports program at the time.

Coach Booth took it upon himself to talk to the administrator at Catholic High. I had been to an interest meeting there with my parents, but had not taken the entrance exam because my dad said there was no way he could afford it. Coach Booth told me that the assistant principal at Catholic High wanted to meet with me and my parents. I was excited, told him thanks, but didn't think it would do any good.

We met with Brother Ronald. I remember sitting in his office because I had been around nuns a lot in elementary school but this was the first time I had ever met a Brother. I still remember the feeling when he said, "I know you didn't take the entrance exam, but we've got your grades from St. Aloysius and we've spoken with the principal and your teachers. We want you to come to school here." He specifically said "want" versus "would like."

The only other thing I remember about that visit was meeting with the choir director to audition to be in the men's choir. I stood next to the piano while Mr. Galliano played and I sang. It was just the two of us and my parents in the room. It felt surreal because just a few hours earlier I had been destined to attend the local public school. I had applied for the magnet school and was number 571 on the waiting list, which I remember because I couldn't imagine that many kids being on the waiting list.

The audition went well, and Mr. G. accepted me into the choir. I thanked Coach Booth for what he had done, but I don't think I truly understood what he had done until years later. He saw in me, as an eighth-grader, what Coach Boudreaux would later pull out of me in my junior and senior years.

One reason I included this story is to properly thank Coach Booth for how he helped change my life. But what he really did was allow himself to be used by God. I know without a doubt that if my chances of getting into the magnet school had been better, there would have been no talk of Catholic High at that point – God made sure I was way down the waiting list. God used Coach Booth and Brother Ronald to give my parents no option but to send me to Catholic High School. God did a miracle that I can never repay him for.

Spring forward to that June day at Christen's house. In the weeks prior to that day I had won the state 3200m on a leg with a stress fracture. Christen was in that race as well. During the race I was boxed in on the first lap. The other competitors knew I was injured and that if they kept me close they had a chance because I had not been able to train for speed in the weeks prior. After a slow first lap Christen realized I was stuck and going well below my desired pace. He moved up next to me to create room and allowed me to get out of the pack. I took off, and the rest, as they say, is history. Christen came in fourth in that race, sacrificing a chance to place higher by giving me the opportunity to run free.

I spent a lot of time with Christen during high school. We ran together and hung out together, so it was nothing new to find myself in his room that day. We started talking about Jesus. Having grown up in a religious family, I knew a lot about God, Jesus, and the Bible. I sang in the choir at mass on Sundays. I considered myself religious. What I learned that day from Christen is that there is a gift that God offers through Jesus to all of us. I don't know if I had missed the knowledge of that gift or if it had never been presented to me until then.

That day I accepted Jesus as my Lord and Savior. Was I immediately a different person in my actions? Nope. In fact there were times you couldn't even tell I was a Christian. It wasn't until years later that I truly understood my decision to accept Jesus. That's when I really began my personal relationship with Christ.

Jesus Christ died on the cross for the sins of mankind. We are all born into sin because of the decision of Adam and Eve to eat the fruit from the tree of knowledge in the Garden of Eden. When the apple was bitten into, mankind fell from the Grace of God into a world of sin where Satan's power is alive. The Old Testament details the struggles of man trying to live up to the life God wants us to have. But no matter how many laws were put in place, no human could repair the damage done to our relationship with God. But every part of the Old Testament points to the coming of Jesus, God Himself coming to earth to finally bring man back to God's true presence.

With Jesus's birth, God came to earth to live among us and show us by example that life without sin is possible. It is easier for us to learn by example and by seeing than it is to simply accept in good faith that something is real or how something is to be done. It is far easier to follow a leader who leads by example. That's what God did when He came to earth as Christ. He had to show us in real life that it is possible to defeat sin in our daily lives. He came to earth to lead us away from sin.

Through the death and resurrection of Jesus, we are now allowed to be in the presence of God through the Holy Spirit. Some people call this your conscience or your moral compass. The Holy Spirit talks to you to try to guide your life to the way God wants you to live. God uses the Holy Spirit to protect you from the dangers of Satan and sin. He also uses other followers of Christ, just as He used them to write the New Testament. While the Old Testament points to Jesus's birth, the New Testament is a road map for how we are to live on this earth.

When you accept Jesus as your Lord and Savior, you begin to understand that the Holy Spirit has been with you all along. There is a spiritual battle going on within you during your time on this earth. The perfect holiness of God does not allow Him to be in the presence of sin. When you choose to sin God is not present, but Satan is. That guilt or remorse you feel after a sinful act is the Holy Spirit returning to you to lead you to repent. This is one reason Christians are misunderstood. Becoming a Christian does not mean you are no longer prone to sin; it simply means you have accepted Jesus and understand that you must ask God for forgiveness for your sinful nature and actions. As a Christian I am still very much a sinner, but I strive daily to live as Christ lived.

* * *

God moved in miraculous ways to introduce me to Jenny. We both attended Texas A&M, and both had the same degree plan. While I was a year ahead of her by class, I didn't start the degree plan until my sophomore year, therefore we had several classes together. In one class with about 400 students

I sat in the back of the lecture hall every time and she sat near the front, and I watched her walk in and sit down in the front for each class. I thought, "There is something about that girl... I have a feeling our paths will cross in some way."

One of my fellow track athletes, Brian, was in one of our smaller classes with us. Jenny sat directly in front of me. She knew Brian from a previous class they had taken together, and they talked from time to time. Neither Jenny nor I recall ever saying a word to each other in that class, as we were both in long-term relationships with other people at the time. Jenny took a much more aggressive approach to finishing college, and graduated ahead of me. One of the requirements for our degree plan was a semester-long internship at a cardiac rehabilitation facility. Jenny interned at a facility in San Antonio, close to her family. Brian interned there as well, and I intended to do the same. After I had turned in my choice of intern site to my instructor, someone else asked if they could have the San Antonio location because her family lived there. Since I had no ties to it I said yes, and moved on to my second choice, which was in Corpus Christi. My grandparents had lived near there before my grandmother passed. My grandfather had moved to Arkansas by that time, but I had always enjoyed visiting the coast.

The time came for me to interview at the facility in Corpus Christi. I didn't realize it at the time, but it was connected to the same doctor's office my grandmother had been to for her heart issues. That's just one way in which God came full circle. I interviewed with the cardiac rehab director, and after the interview she asked if I would like to stay around for a little bit and observe the next patient session. As I waited at the little table in her office, Jenny walked into the room. I thought, "Okay, God, you are obviously telling me something."

A few months later, in January of 1998, I started my internship in Corpus Christi. Jenny was still working there, and I knew instantly that God had put us together... forever. We married in June of 2000 and have enjoyed being best friends ever since.

* * *

In September of 2013 I woke up to my second spontaneous pneumothorax. Since this was the second time, I had to undergo a procedure called pleurodesis in which the inner wall of the rib cage is scarred up so the lung will adhere to it, hopefully preventing a full collapse in the future. During the first day of my hospital stay I couldn't help but wonder why this had happened a second time. God revealed to me in that hospital bed that my life is not about me. I had been far too focused on myself, my family, and the material things of this world. I was active in my church, but my inner thoughts were still of a selfish nature.

My pastor, Grant, came to check on me the second day I was in the hospital. He asked what he could do for me and I told him he could pray for the person in the room next to me. He was puzzled and asked why. I told him I didn't know the person or what their situation was, but there were so many people visiting that they spilled into the hallway and sat on the floor outside the room. The visitors' faces were very sad and emotional. It was obvious that the situation was tough, potentially life and death. I told Grant they needed prayers, not I; that God allowed my lung to collapse the second time because I hadn't responded in the way He wanted me to after the first time. He had to bring me down to that place again to show me that He wanted to use me to help others and not to be so selfish with my life.

Grant went to the white board that the nurses used for notes for each other. He wrote this scripture down:

> *Do nothing out of selfish ambition or vain conceit.*
> *Rather, in humility value others above yourselves, not*
> *looking to your own interests but each of you to the*
> *interests of the others.*
> *— Philippians 2:3-4*

Grant turned back around to look at me and said, "Jerry, this is what you're doing." From that day forward these two verses, in conjunction with a prayer, have shaped every decision I've made.

That hospital stay was also the catalyst for a relationship that changed my life. The other thing God showed me was that I could not live an unselfish life by trying to do it all myself. Satan is too powerful for us to try to be in the middle of the battlefield without someone else to lean on. I reached out to an older man named John from our Bible study group. I knew I needed a more mature Christian to help disciple me, to help me become a stronger Christian, and to hold me accountable for living like Christ. We met weekly for almost two years, and then I found myself in that same hospital, only this time it was John who was hospitalized. He had cancer, which caused a stroke, and a few days later took him from this life to heaven. John taught me how to share Christ with others, not just through words but through actions. I would not be who I am today without John's guidance.

It's been almost five years since my second hospital stay. As I continue to strive to live as Christ-like a life as I can, I have come to the realization that my life is not my own. My life here on earth belongs to God. My purpose is to use the talents He gave me to share Him with others.

If you are struggling to find your significance on this earth and have not trusted in Jesus, I invite you to do so now. Say this quick prayer aloud and open your heart to allow the Holy Spirit to come alive in your life:

Lord, I have sinned against you. I ask you to forgive me. I ask you to lead me and direct my life from this day forward. I accept your son, Jesus, as my personal Savior. I will strive to live my life for you and to share your love with others. Amen.

If you have said this prayer and accepted Jesus, I would like to know about it. Please email me at jerry@allinhealthandwellness.com with the subject "Saved by Grace." My free gift to you is to help you in any way I can as you begin your Christian journey.

Jesus answered, "I am the way and the truth and the life. No one comes to the Father except through me. If you really know me, you will know my Father as well. From now on, you do know him and have seen him.

— John 14:6-7

ABOUT THE AUTHOR

I can do all things through Christ who strengthens me.
– Philippians 4:13

Jerry Snider is the owner of All In Health and Wellness. He graduated from Texas A&M University with a bachelor's degree in exercise physiology in 1998. At Texas A&M he competed on the cross country and track teams, becoming a three-year letterman. He earned certification as a Life Breakthrough Coach from Life Breakthrough Academy in 2016.

Jerry and his wife, Jenny, married in June of 2000 and have lived in Hewitt, Texas, since 2002. They have two children, Abigail and Tai. The Sniders are members of Fellowship Bible Church in Waco, Texas, where they have attended church since 2003. Jerry worked in various businesses and non-profits before opening his business in 2016.

Jerry has volunteered as Sport Performance Coach for Texas Wind Athletics Football since 2016 and helped the team win the first ever Texas Homeschool State Football Championship in 2017. He has served as head coach for the Texas Wind Athletics Track & Field team since 2016 and spent two years as a board member for the organization. He was appointed to the City of Hewitt Parks and Beautification Board in early 2018. He has volunteered in various ways at his church including as usher, speaker at retreats, LIFE group leader, and children's Sunday School leader. Volunteering in his community continues to be very important to him.

In October of 2017 Jerry developed a fundraiser for the City of Hewitt Public Library called All In with Jerry: Running for Readers. He raised $2,000 for the library to expand its selection of books for business owners. To generate awareness for the campaign, Jerry ran every foot of the 258 streets in Hewitt, covering 156 miles in 21 days. He has plans to make this an annual event to continue to support the library.

ABOUT ALL IN HEALTH AND WELLNESS

You must serve only the Lord your God. If you do, I will bless you with food and water, and I will protect you from illness.
— Exodus 23:25

We offer:

- Individualized training plans for runners for distances from 5k to marathon
- Strength and conditioning workouts for high school athletes
- Tailored exercise prescriptions and meal plans

Our focus:

For the everyday person – we teach you to:

- Incorporate the correct amount of exercise into your busy schedule
- Eat healthy foods while eating a "normal" meal plan

For the runner – we prepare you to:

- Finish the race, whether it be a 5k or a marathon
- Be strong physically and mentally

For the athlete – we train you to:

- Be in peak shape for your sport through strength and conditioning
- Achieve your goal of reaching the next level of play

Our strategies:

Tailored coaching to hit your goals

- You set the goal and we coach to it
- Exercise prescriptions and training programs sent via weekly emails

Nutrition guidance

- Basics of a healthy diet included with all programs
- Daily meal plans offered for extra accountability

Realistic workouts

- All exercises can be done from the comfort of your home or in the streets and parks in your neighborhood
- Use principles from plyometrics, isometrics, and calisthenics

Made in the USA
Columbia, SC
30 June 2020